MW00844341

Certified Risk Adjustment Coder (CRC) Exam Study Guide

2018 Edition

Medical Coding Pro

ISBN-13: 978-1987759693
ISBN-10: 1987759699

DEDICATION

To the hard working students preparing for the certification exam. Your work ethic and dedication to the medical coding industry will ensure its health and competency for years to come!

DISCLAIMER AND/OR LEGAL NOTICES:

The information presented herein represents the view of the author as of the date of publication. The book is for informational purposes only.

While every attempt has been made to verify the information provided in this book, neither the author nor his affiliates/partners assume any responsibility for errors, inaccuracies or omissions or for any damages related to use or misuse of the information provided in the book.

Any slights of people or organizations are unintentional. If advice concerning medical or related matters is needed, the services of a fully qualified professional should be sought. Any reference to any person or business whether living or dead is purely coincidental.

SAVE $50! Use Coupon Code "SAVE50"

The Medical Coding Certification Prep Course

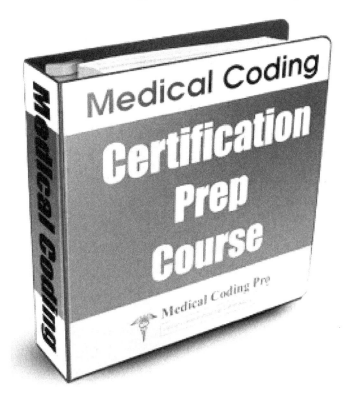

The Medical Coding Certification Prep Course is a web based, self paced, course with over 100 hours of study material. It includes over 700 practice exam questions and answers, 120 Operative Reports, 1,200 terms defined plus current and previous year CPT codes. The course also includes a complete ICD-10 video instruction module, course workbook and one year online access. Professional AAPC approved CPC, CPC-H instructor available to answer questions and give guidance.

For more information go to:

www.MedicalCodingPro.com/medical-coding-certification-prep-course

Dear Customer,

Thank you for your purchase at Medical Coding Pro! We appreciate the trust you have placed in us to help you with your exam preparation.

As a way of showing our appreciation we have created a DVD called "**Exam Passing Secrets**" and we would like to send it to you for **FREE!**

All that we ask is that you email us your feedback that best describes your thoughts on our product. It doesn't matter if the feedback is good or not, we want to hear from you! Your feedback helps a small business like us compete with larger companies by adding a positive review or by telling us how we can improve the product.

Just email us at **freedvd@medicalcodingpro.com** with FREE DVD in the subject line and the following information:

1) The name of the product you purchased.
2) Your product rating on a scale of 1-5, with 5 being the highest.
3) Your feedback. Good feedback might include how our material helped you and what helped you the most.
4) Your full name and shipping address where you would like us to send your FREE DVD.

Thanks again!
Sincerely,

Gregg Zban
Medical Coding Pro

Quick Start Guide

Start by reviewing everything included inside the practice exam bundle. Contents include the following:

1) Medical Coding Exam Strategy
2) Overview
3) Mock Practice Exam Questions & Answers
4) Scoring Sheets
5) Secrets To Reducing Exam Stress
6) Common Anatomical Terminology
7) Medical Terminology Prefixes, Roots, and Suffixes
8) Notes
9) Resources

These resources used properly will give you a good base to prepare for the certification exam.

If you have any questions please email contact us at support@medicalcodingpro.com.

Thank you for your business!

Medical Coding Exam Strategy

One of the first things we should discuss is what "The Strategy" is and what it isn't.

What it is:

A simple, yet powerful, method for increasing your chances of passing the certification exam. Many people have told us that time management was their biggest obstacle in passing the exam. This is what "The Strategy" addresses. It is a road map to pass the exam. It has very little to do with coding knowledge and everything to do with your approach.

What it isn't:

A long, drawn out, hard to follow maze with do's and don'ts reviewing the material that was covered in class. We assume that you know the material, otherwise, it doesn't matter what we teach you the odds are against you.

Why it is important: The reality is many people do not pass the exam the first time. This becomes a costly proposition and one that wasn't bargained for because the next step is an exam retake. The cost: $380. Some even go further and sign up for a three day "boot camp". The cost: about $1200.

Between a rock and a hard place

In this very typical example you passed the Medical Coding class with flying colors but the major hospitals and doctor offices all want a certified medical coder. Why, because it increases their output, makes them more money, and limits their liability for mistakes. So now you're stuck. You have to get certified, but at what cost? It all depends how many times you have to take the certification exam. Follow the steps outlined in "The Strategy" and your next exam could reward you with a certification.

Start by reviewing common mistakes

Some of the most common mistakes made while taking the exam are what we like to call "time wasters". The most important factor to succeeding is time management. You only have 5 hours and 40 minutes to complete the exam (including breaks) and it consists of 150 questions so every minute counts.

The time breakdown goes like this: Exam Time (without breaks) 5 hours 40 minutes or 340 minutes. Exam length: 150 Questions. The easy math is two minute per question. What can we eliminate to save time?

Things Not To Do

1) Answer each question in numerical order.
2) Take too much time on difficult questions first.
3) Read the doctors chart before reading the detail of the question.
4) Not highlighting questions "passed" in the first round

Time Waster #1:

Answering each question in numerical order

If you answer each question in numerical order you will never finish the exam! This is one of the most common mistakes made. If you start out answering the first several questions just fine and then ten questions into the exam you come to a one that you have trouble with, what then? This is a "time burner" and one you can not get hung up on. We will review why this is more important later in "The Strategy".

The Exam is five hours and forty minutes and 150 questions... an average of two minutes per question. The key is to redistribute your time.

Time Waster #2:

Taking too much time on difficult questions the first time through the exam

"The Strategy" is based on a "two pass" system. The first pass is designed to answer the easy questions and highlight the more difficult ones. These will be addressed on the second pass. A good rule of thumb is if you can't answer it in a minute and a half, move on! If you continue to work on these questions you run the risk of not completing the exam or having to rush through the more difficult questions at the end.

Time Waster #3:

Reading the doctors chart before reading the detail of the question

If you get caught in this "time waster" it will rob you of valuable minutes. Always read the question completely before reading the doctors chart. You may be able to eliminate much of the chart because the question is requesting limited information or specific detail.

Time waster #4:

Not highlighting the more difficult questions for the second "pass"

Be prepared. Have a game plan and stick to it. Make sure that you highlight the more difficult questions that you are going to "pass" on in the first round of the exam. If you make the mistake of not highlighting these questions, you will lose valuable minutes trying to search for them in the second round.

Your goal is to answer the easier questions in a minute and a half maximum! Out of 150 questions, let's assume you can answer 60%, or 90 questions, on the first pass averaging 1 minutes per question. That is a total of 135 minutes to answer the first 90 questions. Again, this is an average. That leaves you with 165 minutes to answer the remaining 60 questions. That comes out to 2 minutes per question on the second pass! Now you can be more deliberate with the remaining, more difficult, questions to make sure you answer them correctly.

The "time wasters" have to be minimized or eliminated for you to be successful. Every minute you can save on looking up codes or moving more difficult questions to the second pass the closer you are to your certification.

"Time Wasters" have to be avoided at all costs. Implement a "two pass" system and watch your results increase substantially!

Now let's take an in depth look at the keys that will make all the difference in your exam experience. These are "The Strategy" and "The "Keys" to passing the Medical Coding Certification Exam! These are not difficult, complex strategies. These are straight forward, simple strategies that are easy to implement and highly effective. Follow each step and you will be well on your way to certification.

The Exam Strategy:

1) The basic element of the strategy is making two passes through the exam. The first pass is to answer the questions you can complete in 1 . minute or less. This should be about 60% of the questions. If you can not answer a question in that time, highlight it (mark it for the second pass) and move on! That creates 2 minutes for the remaining 40% which you have identified as more difficult. This should leave you plenty of time on the more difficult questions and improve your overall score.

2) Answer the easier questions in each section on the first pass. You have to answer 70% of the questions or better correctly to pass so answering the easier questions in each section will form a good base of correctly answered questions in all sections thus improving your chances of passing.

3) Identify the first three numbers of the code first. This will help you eliminate answers instantly and narrow your choices for the correct answer. This is a big "time saver". Practice this on your mock practice exam.

4) Read each question before reading the entire doctors chart. Another big "time saver"! Don't waste valuable time reading the entire doctors chart before reading the question. Read the entire question first to find out the specific information the question is requesting.

5) Highlight Procedures one color, Diagnosis another color and Modifiers a third color for quick reference (again, a big time saver!)

The Keys to Success:

Key #1: Study and Preparation.

Don't let anyone fool you into thinking that you don't have to study. That is not the case. You NEED to study, and study hard! The Exam Strategy assumes that you know all the material. There are no shortcuts and The Exam Strategy will only help you pass if you know the material. So put in the time!

One of the best tools available to practice time management for the exam is the Medical Coding Exam System

(www.MedicalCodingExamSystem.com).

It is course dedicated strictly to time management. This will pay big dividends during the exam. We also highly the Faster Coder (www.fastercoder.com) to improve your speed and accuracy. You will quickly find it is worth its weight in gold.

Key #2: Two Complete Passes through the Exam.

During the exam you will be making TWO passes through the entire exam. Let me repeat this because it is at the heart of what we are trying to accomplish. During the exam you will be going through the entire exam twice! The first pass is to answer the easier questions and the second pass is to answer the more difficult ones. Many people do not pass the exam because they get caught up on a few difficult questions and end up not completing the entire exam. You must follow this key element as it is your key to success.

Key #3: Answer The First Pass Questions in 1 1/2 Minutes or Less.

Start the exam by making a first pass. During the first pass answer all the questions that you can complete in a reasonable amount of time (1 1/2 minutes). If you can't answer the question in 1 1/2 minutes highlight it and move on!

Key #4: Highlight All Unanswered Questions in First Pass

If you cannot answer a question within 1 1/2 minutes of the first pass, highlight the unanswered questions in yellow for easy reference during the second pass! Do not forget to highlight them as every second counts and this could be a big time saver!

Key #5: Answer the More Difficult Questions during Second Pass

You should complete the first pass in 135 minutes or less. This will establish a good base of answered questions and leave you with 165 minutes or more to go back and answer the highlighted questions.

Key #6: Do Not Answer the Questions in Order, You Will Fail!

If you take your time and answer the first 80% of questions perfect but run out of time and have to guess on the remaining 20% questions, YOU WILL NOT PASS. You must answer 70% of the questions correctly to pass the exam!

Key #7: Identify the First Three Numbers of the Code

Another good "time saver" is to identify the first three numbers of the code, turn to that page, then go to the sub code numbers.

Key #8: You Can Miss a Certain Percentage in each Section

You can miss a certain percentage in each section and still pass the exam. Your goal is to get enough right to pass. Making two complete passes through the exam will ensures that you are, at minimum, answering the easy questions in each section first. This alone will increase your chances of passing because you will have a base of questions answered in each section. Typically, the last section is rushed through. This will eliminate this hurdle.

Key #9: Read Each Question before Reading the Doctors Chart

Go over each question before you read the doctors chart. This will tell you exactly what you are looking for. You may not need to read the entire chart because the question only references a specific section. This will save you precious time.

Key #10: Highlight Procedures, Diagnosis, and Modifiers

Highlight the patient's treatment/s in different colors for easy reference. I recommend using these colors: Yellow for Procedures, Blue for Diagnosis, and Pink for Modifiers.

Key #11: You Must Answer 70% correctly to pass the exam

You must keep moving! Leave the tough questions and move on. Ask around to anyone who did not pass the exam the first time (or more) and see what they say. It's all about time management and using the right tips and techniques. So to that end, if you do not follow any other advice, follow this! Do the easiest questions first.

Bonus Tips:

1) Eliminate any answers that begin with an E-Code instantly! Cross it out... this will reduce your selection of answers.

2) Code injections with an administration charge.

3) Supervision and Interpretation components require physician supervision. In radiology procedures this means the radiologist has participated.

4) Know the difference between modifier 26 and modifier TC from your HCPCS II book.

5) Diabetes mellitus – etiology code first then the manifestation code.

6) Trauma accident- always code the most severe injury first

7) Tab all your books including CPT, HCPCS Level II, ICD-10-CM, for quick reference.

8) Code burns on the depth of the burn (1st, 2nd, or 3rd degree). Burns are classified to the extent of the body surface involved. When coding burns of multiple sites, assign separate codes for each burn site. Also burns of the same local site (three-character category level, T20-T28), but of different degrees should be coded to the highest degree documented.

9) Multiple fractures, code by site and sequence by severity.

10) If the same bone is fractured or dislocated, code the fracture only.

11) If the question doesn't state open or closed fracture, code as a closed fracture.

12) Late effects (now called "sequela); is a residual of previous illness or injury. Code the residual and then the cause. Reference "late" in the index.

13) Sequence symptoms first if no diagnosis.

14) Study Medicare A, B, C, D

15) Understand modifier 62 co-surgeons (look on exam for surgeon A and B)

16) ***KEEP MOVING, KEEP MOVING, AND KEEP MOVING!***

Overview

The Certified Risk Adjustment Coder (CRC) Exam

- 150 multiple-choice questions (proctored)

- 5 hours and 40 minutes to finish the exam

- 1 free retake

- $380 ($300 AAPC Students)

- Open code book (manuals)

The CRC examination consists of questions regarding the correct application of ICD-10-CM diagnosis codes used for risk adjustment coding.

The CRC® exam thoroughly covers:

Compliance
Diagnosis Coding
Documentation Improvement
Pathophysiology/ Medical Terminology/ Anatomy
Purpose and Use of Risk Adjustment Models
Quality Care
Risk Adjustment Models

Mock Practice Exam Questions & Answers 2017 Edition

The following is a Medical Coding Pro mock practice exam. You may not use any outside materials for this exam other than the manuals referenced by the American Academy of Professional Coders (AAPC ©).

The code research program we use and recommend is Find A Code. You can locate it at: www.findacode.com?pc=MEDCOPRO.

To pass the certification exam you must manage your time carefully. If after going through this practice you determine that time management is a skill you may need additional assistance with, the Medical Coding Exam System (www.MedicalCodingExamSystem.com) is an excellent resource for additional support.

If you want additional resources to prepare for the certification exam we highly recommend FasterCoder.com (www.FasterCoder.com).

Mock CRC Exam - 150 Questions

Compliance - 24 Questions

1. The purpose of RADV audits are to _____.

a. Find providers who are exploiting Medicare guidelines by CMS
b. Make sure providers are not under coding or over coding
c. Recoup improper payments under Medicare Part C
d. Both A and C

2. Which of the following is an acceptable provider to submit diagnosis for RAPS?

a. Ophthalmologist & Medical Assistant
b. CNA
c. Internist
d. None of the above are correct

3. Electronically signed and authenticated by Mary Hernandez, MDFAC is an acceptable signature.

a. True
b. False

4. The diagnosis codes (_____, and _____) have been adopted under HIPAA for all healthcare settings.

a. ICD-10 and CPT codes
b. Tabular List and Alphabetic Index
c. CPT Codes and HCPCS codes
d. ICD-10 and HCPCS codes

5. When a guideline requires that a linkage between two conditions be explicitly documented, provider documentation does not have to link the conditions to code them as related.

a. True
b. False

6. If upon conducting an internal review of submitted diagnosis codes, the plan sponsor must determine that any diagnosis codes that have been submitted do not meet risk adjustment submission requirements, the plan sponsor is responsible for:

a. Deleting the submitted diagnosis codes
b. Discussing the errors with providers
c. Ignoring the diagnosis, that does not meet requirements
d. Receiving and reconciling the reports in a timely matter

7. To purposely bill for services that were never given or to bill for service that has a higher reimbursement than the service provided is called _____.

a. HIPAA
b. Fraud and Abuse
c. HITECH
d. Both A and B are correct

8. What are the benefits of a compliance plan:

a. Imprisonment up to 5 years for offenders
b. More accurate payments of claims
c. Less chance of violating self- referral and anti-kickback statues
d. Both B and C are correct

9. CMS can use standardized bids as _____ payments to plans because of risk adjusting plan bids.

a. Final
b. Base
c. Duplicate
d. First

10. Medicare is a federal health insurance program administered by the

a. CMS
b. United States of America
c. HIPPA
d. Both A and C are correct

11. Match the following Medicare programs

Part A	Prescription Drug Coverage
Part C	Inpatient hospitals, skilled facilities, hospice and home health
Part D	Combined benefits of Part A and Part B
Part B	Physicians services, outpatient care & preventative services

a. Part A=Inpatient hospitals, skilled facilities, hospice and home health, Part B= Physicians services, outpatient care & preventative services, Part C= Combined benefits of Part A and Part B, D= Prescription drug coverage.

b. Part B=Inpatient hospitals, skilled facilities, hospice and home health, Part D= Physicians services, outpatient care & preventative services, Part A= Combined benefits of Part A and Part B, C= Prescription drug coverage.

c. Part A=Inpatient hospitals, skilled facilities, hospice and home health, Part C= Physicians services, outpatient care & preventative services, Part D= Combined benefits of Part A and Part B, C= Prescription drug coverage.

12. Which system contains the diagnostic data submitted by Medicare Advantage plans, PACE organizations and cost plans?

a. CMS
b. HPMS
c. RAPS
d. NMUD

13. CMS requires Medicare Advantage plans to collects risk data from which organization for calculation of the risk score for use in the payment calculation and payment reconciliation?

a. Hospice
b. In/Outpatient Hospitals, Physician
c. Physicians
d. Inpatient and Outpatient hospitals

14. It is acceptable to code from which of the following?

a. History
b. Quest Lab results
c. CT scan
d. CNA note

15. Echocardiogram Report

Patient Name: John Smith
Referring Physician: Ron Ramnath MD

Technique: Echo was performed conforming to the American Society of Echocardiography protocols for a complete study using 2D/ M-Mode, spectral and color flow doppler modalities in obtaining imagine, hemodynamics measurements and calculations.

Physician Review:
Conclusion:

1. Normal LV size and function
2. Left ventricular ejection fraction estimated by 2D at 35-40%
3. Normal right ventricle abnormal 45mmHg consistent with severe pulmonary hypertension.

Report the appropriate codes:

a. I27.20
b. I11.0, I27.20
c. I10
d. None of the above

16. CMS requires the treating provider to sign the medical record in a timely matter within _____ days.

a. 30 days
b. 60 days
c. 90 days
d. 120 days

17. The RADV audits are conducted by?

a. NCQA
b. HIPAA
c. CMS
d. OSHA

18. What information is identified during a RADV audit?

a. Frequent visits
b. Collection history
c. All diagnosis codes reported are supported in the medical record
d. Referral to specialist as needed

19. In an HRADV/ IVA identifies which of the following?

a. DOS that supports HCC's (through diagnosis codes)
b. Verification for the enrollment status
c. Claim system accuracies verifications
d. All of the above are correct

20. Which provider is more than likely be subjected to a targeted RADV audit?

a. Providers who have had problematic audits in the past.
b. Plans who have higher risk scores when compared to fee for service Medicare.
c. Providers who have complaints of fraud and abuse.
d. Both A and B

21. Which of the following statements is NOT true:

a. CMS RADV is typically two to three years after payment; while HHS HRADV occurs typically six months after year end.

b. CMS RADV allows up to five best records to support an HCC.

c. Clinicians in an ACO are held accountable for the quality.

d. CMS RADV typically involves approximately 45 health plans.

22. Which concept is a responsive to FFS (fee-for- service) payment?

a. ASO
b. HHS
c. ADRAV
d. CMS

23. CMS has established 33 nationally recognized measures in four key domains in which to measure the quality of care provided by Accountable Care Organizations (ACO's). What are the four Domains?

a. Patient/ Caregiver Experience, Care Coordination/ Patient Safety, Preventative Health, At-Risk Population.

b. Heart Failure, Care Coordination/ Patient Safety, Preventative Health, At-Risk Population.

c. Patient/ Caregiver Experience, Diabetes Measures/ Patient Safety, Preventative Health, At-Risk Population.

d. Patient/ Caregiver Experience, Care Coordination/ Patient Safety, Hypertension Measures, At-Risk Population.

24. Provider document chronic kidney disease stage I, chronic kidney stage II, chronic kidney stage III. Which action should be taken:

a. Code lowest stage
b. Code to the severity
c. Code neither diagnosis
d. Query provider to confirm the stage

Diagnosis Coding - 63 Questions

25. A 42-year-old Female presents to the office today with history of Uncontrolled Type 2 Diabetes which was unable to be controlled with Metformin. At the last visit patient was prescribed Novolog 10 units twice daily however, patient states she refuses to continue to inject herself with a needle every day. Patient is fully aware of the harm this may cause to her body. What are the correct diagnosis to report for this encounter?

a. Z79.4, E11.9
b. E11.65, E11.9, Z79.4, Z91.128
c. E11.65, Z91.128, Z79.4, E11.9
d. E11.65, Z79.4, Z91.128

26. 35-year-old HIV positive male was seen in ED for gunshot wound to lower back. Which are the correct diagnosis to submit for encounter?

a. Z21, S31.000A, M54.5
b. S31.000D, M54.5
c. S31.000A, B20
d. S31.000D, B20

27. 52-year-old female presents with left side weakness S/P CVA 2 days ago. Patient also complains of lower back and wrist pain starting without injuries about 1 month ago. She has been wearing a back brace, taking Methotrexate for her arthritis in her wrist and pain is not improving. Feels sore, achy, and has moderate sharp pain at times when she moves her wrist.

PT ADMITS: numbness/ tingling, increasing pain.

DENIES: redness, no Hx of injury or trauma no new injury.

CURRENT MEDICATIONS REVIEWED & RECONCILED: -Crestor 10mg - Methotrexate -furosemide 40mg -Sertraline 60mg -lisinopril 2.5 mg - ibuprofen 800 mg -Lantus 100u- Vit B 12- Keppra

PAST MEDICAL HISTORY INCLUDES: Seizure disorder (Grand Mal), RA, HTN

EXAMINATION: Wrist/Hand: INSPECTION: Left wrist, no swelling, no redness, no ecchymosis, no deformity RANGE OF MOTION: F R O M PALPATION: TTP radial styloid, no tenderness to palpation on ulna, radiocarpal joint, scaphoid… STRENGTH: normal grip, normal strength of flexors and extensors NEUROVASCULAR EXAM: 5/5 strength and normal sensation radial, median, and ulnar nerve distribution TINNEL'S SIGN: Negative PHALEN'S SIGN: Negative FINKELSTEIN'S TEST: Negative VASCULAR: No vascular compromise, skin warm and dry

ASSESSMENT/ PLAN –
Stroke- continue to take baby aspirins twice daily for the next month until follow up with me.

Neuropathy due to Vitamin B12 deficiency- new Rx for gabapentin and hold vitamin b12 until next follow up Vitamin B levels are elevated.
Thrombocytopenia- resolved; Platelets are low

VITAL SIGNS: Ht. 72, Wt. 278.2, BMI 44.17, BP 106/64, HR 72, RR 16, Pain constant 5.

Choose the correct coding diagnosis:

a. I69.354, M06.032, G40.409, I10, E53.8, G63, Z68.44
b. I69.354, M06.032, G40.409, I10, E53.8, G63, Z68.41
c. I63.9, M06.032, R56.9, I10, G63, E53.8, D69.6
d. I63.9, M06.4, R56.9, I10, G63, E53.8

28. The patient has acute Thrombosis with long term anticoagulant. Code the condition.

a. I82.409, Z79.01
b. Z79.4, I82.403
c. I82.409, Z79.4
d. Z79.01, I82.409

29. Patient presents with chest wall pain, possibly angina. Patient has ASHD s/p CABG. Physician confirms angina from stress test and prescribes patient nitroglycerine PRN. Code the diagnosis.

a. I25.700
b. I25.10, I20.9
c. I25.119, Z95.1
d. I25.119

30. Patient present with unstageable pressure ulcer on the left buttocks. Code the diagnosis.

a. L89.000
b. L40.1
c. L89.319
d. L89.320

31. Use chart below to answer the following question:

CMS-HCC DISEASE HIERARCHIES

If the Disease Group is Listed in This Column...		...Then Drop the Associated Disease Group(s) Listed in This Column	
HCC Disease group	Label	HCC Disease group	Label
17	Diabetes with Ketoacidosis	18, 19	Diabetes with/ without complications
18	Diabetes with Chronic Conditions	19	Diabetes w/o complications

Patient presents in the ED with Ketoacidosis due to DM. Patient has a history of DM II w/ CKD and DM with neuropathy. Pertaining to the guidelines above which is the correct reporting code?

a. E10.10
b. E11.69, E11.22, E11.42
c. E11.9, E11.22, E11.10
d. E13.00, E11.22, E11.42

32. 70-year-old with COPD is admitted to the hospital with severe sepsis caused by acute respiratory failure. What diagnosis code(s) should be reported?

a. J96.00, J45.901
b. R65.20, N17.9, J96.00
c. N17.9, J96.00 R65.20
d. R65.20

33. Patient presents at the cardiologist for a follow up of his hypertension and CKD IV. Both conditions are uncontrolled and medication had to be increased. What code(s) should be reported?

a. I10
b. I11.0
c. I11.0, N18.4
d. I12.9, N18.4

34. Which statement(s) is/ are true regarding ICD-10?

a. Diagnosis codes drives the risk scores

b. The codes do not describe the service performed, just patients medical condition

c. Stands for International Classification of Diseases -10th Edition- Clinical Modifications

d. All the above are correct

35. 32-year-old Female diagnosed with emergency hypertension. Select the diagnosis code.

a. I11.0
b. I16.1
c. I12.9
d. I10

36. A patient presents to the emergency room complaining of migraine headaches and nausea. A CT scan was ordered and patient was diagnosed with migraine with aura and fatigue. The correct codes are:

a. R11.0, G43.111
b. G43.119, R11.0
c. G43.119, R53.83
d. R53.82, G43.111

37. When does a late effect occur:

a. Immediately
b. Months later
c. Years later
d. All the above are correct

38. Based on the general coding guidelines for sequela (late effects) select the appropriate codes.

a. M81.8 Other osteoporosis without current pathological fracture/ E64.8 Sequelae of other nutritional deficiencies (calcium deficiency).

b. I69.351 Hemiplegia and hemiparesis following cerebral infarction affecting right dominant side.

c. None of the above.

d. Both A and B are correct.

39. A patient is treated for hyperlipidemia and hypertension. Determine the correct diagnosis codes.

a. I12.9, E78.2
b. E78.5, I10
c. R03.0, I11.0
d. E78.00, I10

40. Patient is seen in physician's office and diagnosed with hypertension caused by HFpEF.

a. I11.0, I50.32
b. I10, I50.31
c. I11.0, I50.9
d. I10, I50.9

41. Patient is diagnosed with systolic heart failure due to hypertension and CKD stage V.

a. N18.4, I12.9, I50.9
b. I50.22, N18.5
c. I13.2, N18.5, I50.22
d. I13.0, N18.4, I50.9

42. Varicose veins are found where in the ICD-10- CM?

a. Category I82.-
b. Category I83.-
c. Category H82.-
d. Category H83.-

43. ICD-10-CM equates pressure ulcers to _____.

a. Bed sores
b. Decubitus and plastic
c. Pressure area and pressure sores
d. All of the above are correct

44. How many characters are required when coding all pressure ulcers?

a. Five
b. Four
c. Six
d. Seven

45. The proper code for Age-related Osteoporosis with current pathological fracture, right humerus , subsequent encounter for fracture with routine healing.

a. M80.021A
b. M80.021D
c. M80.021G
d. M80.021K

46. Patient came in for follow up for CKD IV, ESRD and hyperparathyroidism. Patient is stable and managed well with dialysis on Tuesdays and Thursdays for 4 hours. Select the diagnosis:

a. N18.6, Z99.2
b. N18.4, N25.81, Z79.1
c. N25.81, N18.4
d. N18.6, N25.81, Z99.2

47. A patient who undergoes a kidney transplant may continue to have Chronic Kidney Disease.

a. True
b. False

48. Patient diagnosed with pressure ulcers on each cheek of buttocks. Select the diagnosis:

a. L89.000
b. L89.312, L89.311
c. L89.329, L89.319
d. L89.329

49. Which of the following are sequenced accurately?

a. L89.222, L89.623
b. N18.3, I12.9
c. L89.623, L89.222
d. L89.221,L89.623

50. Patient presents in the office complaining of painful inflammation of his right buttocks. The provider performs an exam of his right buttocks and diagnoses the patient with Cellulitis of the right buttocks. Select the diagnosis:

a. L03.312
b. L03.311
c. L03.317
d. L03.313

51. Cellulitis can be found in what chapter in the ICD-10-CM book?

a. 8th Chapter
b. 12th Chapter
c. 10th Chapter
d. 4th Chapter

52. Disease and disorders of the skin and subcutaneous includes which of the following?

a. Nails
b. Hair, Hair Follicles
c. Sweat Glands
d. All the above are correct

53. Using the hierarchy table provided, which HCC is ultimately utilized for patient diagnosed with CKD stage 5 w/ dialysis treatment and Acute Renal Failure on discharge from Hospital.

If this HCC is found ...	Disease Group Label	Then drop these HCCs:
135	Acute Renal Failure	136, 137
136	Chronic Kidney Disease 5	137
134	Dialysis Status	135, 136, 137
137	Chronic Kidney Disease	

a. 134
b. 136 and 134
c. 135
d. 136

54. Which are examples of 2016/17 Medicare advantage HCC Category?

a. Substance Abuse
b. Transplants
c. Metabolic
d. All of the above

55. A patient present with fatigue, vomiting, and back pain. The provider documents the symptoms are consistent acute gastritis. Select the diagnosis.

a. R11.2, R10.9
b. K29.70
c. K29.71
d. K29.90

56. Assign the appropriate ICD-10-CM code(s). Primary lung cancer metastatic to the liver.

a. C34.90, C76.0
b. C32.8, C78.00
c. C78.00
d. C34.90, C78.7

57. Patient present at the office with Obesity, HTN, COPD CKD IV. Coder reported E66.01, I12.9 N18.4 and J44.9. Which code should NOT have been reported?

a. I12.9
b. E66.01
c. N18.4
d. E11.9

58. **History of Present Illness**

Patient presenting for evaluation of Pain in the sacroiliac joint. Injury occurred while at rest, no known injury. Onset of symptoms was 4 months ago. Patient reports pain is 10/10 in severity.   Symptomatic treatment prior to arrival includes ice, heat, Tylenol/Ibuprofen, codeine. All other systems reviewed and negative except as stated above in the HPI.

Past medical history: COPD, DM, neuropathy in Vitamin 12.
No allergies.

Medications Includes: Metformin, Novolog Insulin 30/60
Tobacco use: Daily Smoker 2-4 packs per day
Alcohol Use: No

PHYSICAL EXAM:
Constitutional: No acute distress
Vital signs and nursing notes reviewed
HEENT: Atraumatic norm cephalic
CV: Well perfused
Respiratory: wheezing and cough (due to smoking)
Abdomen: Nondistended
Back: No obvious deformities; sacroiliitis
Skin: Normal color, warm and dry
Wrist Examination: normal hand/wrist exam, no swelling, tenderness, instability. Ligaments intact, FROM all joints, scaphoid (snuffbox) tenderness present
Neuro: Oriented x3, numbness and tingling, no sensation

Medical Decision Making
Patient presenting with ***. Presentation consistent with carpal tunnel syndrome. Radiographs were not ordered as there was no history of trauma. Provided wrist splint. Symptomatic treatment was discussed. Patient may use ibuprofen/Tylenol as needed for pain. Follow up with primary physician or orthopedic clinic if continued pain. Return to office if pain uncontrolled, neurovascular change, or other concerns.

Impression:
Carpal Tunnel Syndrome
Back and wrist pain
Neuropathy

Code all the appropriate codes even if codes are not mapped.

a. M46.1, J44.9, E11.42, J41.0, M25.539, M54.9, G62.0
b. M25,539, M54.9, G62.0
c. M46.1, J44.9, E11.9, G63, E53.9, J41.0, Z79.4, G56.00
d. E11.42, J41.0, M54.9, M25.539

59. Which statement(s) is/are TRUE:

a. If in the assessment section of an EMR states Diabetes – E11.9 then E11.9 should be coded.

b. If in the assessment section of an EMR record states Diabetes with CKD 3 then E11.43 should be coded

c. In the assessment section of an EMR record states HTN (I12.9) Smokers cough (J41.0) ESRD (N18.6) then I12.9, N18.6, J41 should be coded.

d. If in the assessment section of an EMR records states Major depression (F33.41) then F33.41 should be coded.

a. Both C and D are correct
b. Both A and B are correct
c. Both A and C are correct
d. Both B and C are correct

60. Patient diagnosed with major depression recurrent mild. What is the appropriate code?

a. F32.0
b. F33.41
c. F33.40
d. F33.0

61. Patient diagnosed with metastatic cancer of the left ovary. What is the appropriate code?

a. C79.62
b. C79.31
c. C79.51
d. C81.03

62. Patient diagnosed with neuropathy due to Albinism. How would you code this?

a. G63
b. G62.9, G63, E07.00
c. E70.319, G63
d. G65.0

63. Patient diagnosed with carcinoma in situ of vulva. What is the appropriate code.

a. D07.1
b. C51.0
c. D70.0
d. C51.9

64. Patient present with a severe cough onset two days ago. CXR was ordered and confirmed diagnosis of COPD was found. Patient was prescribed Proair and was instructed to follow up if symptoms get worse after three days. Patient was counseled on smoking and is aware of risks of continuously smoking.

Coder has reported J44.9, R05. Which code should have ALSO been reported?

a. J41.0
b. Z87.891
c. F17.210
d. F17.211

65. Patient presents to ER with foot contusion. While grooming his horse at the ranch, the horse stepped on his left foot. Select the appropriate codes:

a. S90.32XA, W55.19XA, Y93.K3
b. S90.32XA
c. W55.19XA, Y93.K3
d. S90.32XD

66. Which is the correct code for a benign neoplasm of larynx?

a. D14.4
b. D14.2
c. D16.00
d. D14.1

67. Which Is the correct code for Moderate protein calorie malnutrition?

a. E43
b. E46
c. E42
d. E44.0

68. A patient is admitted after being found in his car unresponsive at his place of employment. The patient had left-sided hemiparesis from a previous stroke. The physician documents current CVA as the final diagnosis and the patient is discharged home. What ICD-10-CM code(s) should be reported?

a. I63.9
b. I69.959, I69.9
c. I63.9, I69.954
d. I69.954, I63.9

69. A patient is coming in for follow up of his Atrial fibrillation hypertension and cardiomyopathy. Both conditions are stable, and he is told to continue with his medications. What ICD-10-CM code(s) should be reported?

a. I48.2
b. I11.9, I43, I48.92
c. I48.91, I11.9 I42.9
d. I48.91, I11.9, I43

70. A 42-year-old male presents to the office with history of ongoing diabetes which has been uncontrolled even with insulin for follow-up exam. During this encounter the physician notes a chronic diabetic wound of his right foot and determines acute osteomyelitis. After examination and testing the family practice physician recommends the gentleman to be seen by a general surgeon for treatment of his osteomyelitis of his right foot or an amputation of right foot. What are the correct diagnoses to report for this encounter?

a. E11.65, I96
b. Z79.4, E11.9, M86.172
c. E11.65, M86.172, Z79.4, Z79.891
d. E11.65, M86.171, Z79.4

71. Internal medicine has asked me to see the patient for consideration of further intervention. The patient is known to have hypertension. There is no history of diabetes or hyperlipidemia. He is status post parathyroidectomy. Status post inguinal hernia repair. He is allergic to PENICILLIN (the patient believes he had a rash to penicillin, although it was so many years ago that he cannot accurately recall).

Current Medications:
Aspirin 325 mg p.o. qd., metformin 16 mg p.o. qd., Aciphex 20mg p.o. bid.

The patient is married and was accompanied with his wife. He is a construction worker and works as a repairman for Total Plumbing. He does not smoke. A review of systems was reviewed and are all-negative except for above. These records are in his inpatient record dated 03/05/2017.

The patient is a healthy-appearing man who appeared younger than 70. He was afebrile. P 70 and electrocardiogram monitor showed that he was in normal sinus rhythm.

Vitals: B/P is 160/70, Ht 171cm, Wt 75 kg.
ROS: Lungs were clear to auscultation. Heart tones normal. Examination of his abdomen was negative. His extremities were normal with normal dorsalis pedis pulses bilaterally. There was no cervical bruit audible. There was no gross neurologic deficit.

Impression:
Severe headaches, Hypertension.

Based on the documentation provided, which diagnosis are reported for risk adjustment purposes?

a. E11.9
b. E11.9, E78.5, I10
c. E89.2
d. E89.2, I10

72. Patient presents to the medical office today for follow up of MRI of the brain, with a high fever of 101 and shakes. Patient has a history of CVA, HTN and Cerebral Palsy.

Medication reviewed:
Metformin 500mg QID
Diazepam qd
Lisinopril

Patient has a blood pressure of 200/150. Sent patient to the hospital possible heart attack in office. MRI showed to be remarkable except for calcification of the basal ganglia and Empty Sella.

Based on the documentation provided, which diagnosis are reported for risk adjustment purposes?

a. I36.0, E11.9, I10, I25.2
b. G80.9, G23.8, E23.6
c. G23.8, E11.9, I10,
d. I21.01, I36.0, G80.9, E11.9

73. Code Neuropathy caused by Oxycodone

a. G62.0
b. G63, F11.20
c. F11.20, G62.1
d. G62.0, T40.2X5D

74. Which of the following Acute codes could be coded once the patient has been discharged from the hospital?

a. I63.00
b. I21.3
c. E13.10
d. K56.690

75. Brackets [ ] are used in the tabular list to enclose

a. Synonyms, alternate words
b. Explanatory phrases
c. Main terms
d. Both A and B are correct

76. Which is the correct code for sickle cell anemia?

a. D57.20
b. D57.1
c. D57.412
d. D57.40

77. Patient presents for a follow up of fatigue fracture of lumbar vertebra two years ago. What is the appropriate code to report?

a. M84.40XA
b. M48.41XD
c. M48.40XA
d. M48.46XS

78. What is the ICD-10-CM code for male right sided breast cancer?

a. C50.921
b. C50.929
c. C50.911
d. No ICD-10 code for male breast cancer

79. The 4th character in an ICD-10-CM code further defines:

a. The site
b. Etiology
c. Manifestations or state of disease/ conditions
d. All of the above

80. What are the ICD-10-CM codes for Endocarditis caused by a Q fever?

a. A78, I39
b. I39, A78
c. I38, A78
d. A78, I40.0

81. What is the ICD-10-CM code for Chronic Pulmonary Embolism managed by Coumadin anticoagulant?

a. Z79.01, I27.82
b. I27.82
c. I27.20
d. I27.82, Z79.01

82. Code for bilateral shoulder pain.

a. M25.851, M25.852
b. M25.861, M25.862
c. M25.551, M25.552
d. M25.511, M25.512

83. There can be more than one way to find the correct code. For example, to find COPD you could also locate it under:

a. Obstruction/ lung/ disease/ chronic
b. Disease/ lung/ obstruction
c. Disease/ pulmonary / chronic obstruction
d. All of the above

84. In the outpatient setting, it is OK to code the following example of languages found in medical records.

a. Rule out
b. Certain
c. Suspected
d. Probable

85. Diagnosis: Fatigue, suspected iron deficiency anemia.

a. R53.83
b. R53.83, D50.9
c. E61.1
d. E61.1, D58.2

86. A patient presents with severe chest pain, abdominal pain, nausea and vomiting. The provider diagnoses patient with acute appendicitis. What is/ are the ICD-10-CM code(s) to report?

a. K35.89
b. R10.9
c. R10.9, K35.80
d. K35.80

87. Patient is admitted to the hospital with fatigue and coughing up blood. Patient is being worked up to rule out HIV vs Tuberculosis. Which are the appropriate codes to report?

a. A15.9, B20
b. R53.82, R04.2
c. A15.9
d. Both B and C are correct

Documentation Improvement - 18 Questions

88. 75-year-old male seen in the office today for a follow up on history of prostate cancer. No symptoms now and currently on Lupron. Which of the following is the best action?

a. Code Z85.46
b. Code C61, and advise provider to change to active prostate cancer at next visit.
c. Code C61.2
d. Recommend provider to update history of Prostate Cancer to Active Prostate Cancer because patient is on treatment.

89. What is translating medical documentation into codes?

a. Interpreting Coding
b. Risk Adjustment Coding
c. Medical Coding
d. None of the above are correct

90. Mild CKD stage 2 code N18.2, which is true?

a. R/o N18.4
b. Assessment and Plan: Moderate CKD
c. Assessment and Plan: Dialysis status
d. A/P Mild CKD

91. Which of the following is NOT appropriate to assign ICD-10 code J44.9?

a. COPD
b. Chronic Obstructive Asthma
c. Asthmatic Bronchitis Chronic
d. Chronic Bronchitis

92. What are risk factors?

a. Anatomy about a condition
b. Acute and Chronic conditions
c. Life coverage and medical history
d. Notes about patients known medical history or social habits that may place the patient at risk to develop a condition.

93. Why is it important to document everything on the progress note?

a. Helps identify those patients who may have a higher medical need than others.
b. Help coders bill more
c. Help patients pay less
d. To avoid an audit

94. A patient has been complaining of chronic pain in the left leg. Physician examines the patient's leg and is diagnosed with R side leg pain Sciatica. Select the appropriate diagnosis:

a. M54.32
b. M54.2
c. M54.31
d. Recommend confirming the correct site of sciatica

95. Medical documentation reviews are used to forecast future health needs, while explaining current needs and expenses.

a. True
b. False

96. Which two are most important when coding?

a. Patient name and signatures
b. Providers signatures and credentials
c. Patient name and date of birth
d. Patient name and history

97. Which are acceptable signatures?

a. Signature stamped
b. "Finalized by"
c. "Signed but not read"
d. "Dictated but not read or reviewed"

98. J44.9 stable, continue meds. E11.42; controlled, labs ordered.

Select the statement which makes the above statements true.

a. Coders can report if signed by provider
b. It is mandatory to use ICD10 codes instead of words written
c. Reporting the diagnosis code alone is not appropriate documentation
d. COPD is equal to J44.9. It is ok to report J44.9 because physicians are coders.

99. Which of the following diagnosis can be coded without documentation in a medical record?

a. CHF
b. CVA / Stroke
c. Multiple Sclerosis
d. Both A and C are correct

100. A diabetic patient presents with an ulcer on the greater left big toe. The ulcer requires cleaning and re-bandaging. Which conditions should the coder report?

a. Diabetes
b. Ulcer of the toe
c. Diabetes and the ulcer of the greater left big toe
d. Diabetes manifestation and the ulcer of the left greater toe

101. Which of the following can coder assign history codes?

a. History of DVT, no longer on coumadin.
b. History of Smokers Cough, continues smoking, hypoxemia utilize home O2 daily.
c. History ESRD, Transplant status.
d. History of breast cancer undergoing chemotherapy.

102. Which is NOT used to capture current diagnosis codes?

a. Exam
b. Past Medical History
c. Radiology reports
d. Assessment and Plan

103. Select the codes that can be assumed to have a cause and effect relationship between both diagnosis codes that are reported for the same encounter.

a. Hypertension and CHF
b. Hypertension and CKD
c. COPD and DM
d. Both A and B are correct

104. Which is NOT appropriate for documentation on a medical record to be reported?

a. Arrows pointed up or down
b. Probable/ Suggestive diagnosis/ Confirmed
c. Rule out HIV
d. A and C

105. Which of the following statements are true?

a. Providers must understand how risk adjustment models work and the models' purposes.
b. The reporting of all diagnosis is important to establish the right risk adjustment factors.
c. HRADV is conducted annually
d. All of the above

Pathophysiology/ Medical Terminology/ Anatomy - 9 Questions

106. What is the function of the kidneys?

a. Filter the blood to remove waste and produce urine
b. Drain urine from the Urethra
c. Maintain the homeostasis of water, ions.
d. Both A and C are correct.

107. Which statement is true:

a. COPD is reversible
b. COPD affects your lungs and ability to breathe.
c. COPD is primarily caused by smoking, and damage to your lungs can't be reversed.
d. Both B and C are correct.

108. Emphysema is the disease of

a. Alveoli
b. Bronchioles
c. Trachea
d. Capillaries

109. Which cavity is the heart located and what is its function?

a. Thoracic Cavity; Provide blood and nutrients to body tissues by transporting the oxygen throughout the body.

b. Thoracic Cavity; Provide oxygen and nutrients to body tissues by transporting the blood throughout the body.

c. Dorsal Cavity; Provide oxygen and nutrients to body tissues by transporting the blood throughout the body.

d. Dorsal Cavity; Provide blood and nutrients to body tissues by transporting the oxygen throughout the body.

110. The pharynx, larynx, and trachea are part of what system?

a. Digestive
b. Respiratory
c. Urinary
d. Upper Respiratory

111. How many layers is the heart composed of:

a. Four
b. Two
c. Three
d. Five

112. Using the words heart, muscle and disease, translate for the medical term.

a. Cardi/o, my/o, pathy
b. Cardio/o, marrow, plasty
c. Phleb/o, Cyst/o, pathy
d. None of the above

113. What are the two parts that comprise the nervous system?

a. Spine and nerves
b. Brain and spinal cord
c. Brain and spinal cord, and nerves
d. Nerves and brain

114. Which ventricle side of the heart is smaller and why?

a. The muscle surrounding the left ventricle is stronger and larger that of the right ventricle, because the left side is responsible for pumping the blood throughout the entire body.

b. The right-side ventricle is larger because the left ventricle must pump blood throughout partial of the body.

Purpose and Use of Risk Adjustment Models - 12 Questions

115. What is the purpose of Risk Adjustment?

a. To allow CMS to pay plans for the risk of the beneficiaries they enroll.
b. A random audit is a selected group of documentation notes selected by a random doctor.
c. Document all clinical finding in the medical records and submit for reimbursements.
d. All the above are correct.

116. Health risk is re-determined every year. HCCs must be captured how often?

a. Every 6 months
b. Every 12 months
c. Every 24 months
d. Every 12 Weeks

117. Segments of the ESRD models include:

a. Dialysis
b. Transplant
c. Post- Graft/ Functioning graft
d. All of the answers are correct

118. Qualified physician data for risk adjustment does not require a face to face visit.

a. True
b. False

119. Which model diagnosis does not count toward the risk score?

a. Retrospective Models
b. Current Models
c. ESRD and Rxx Models
d. Future Models

120. Which of the following statements are true?

a. Not all ICD codes carry value in risk adjustment models.
b. Substance abuse, complications and HTN are all examples of HCC categories.
c. Infections, Neoplasms and Diabetes are all examples of HCC categories.
d. Both A and C

121. Reviews that will affect the next year and not the current year are called

a. Concurrent
b. Prospective
c. Skilled
d. Retrospective

122. Ongoing reviews are called:

a. Prospective
b. Retrospective
c. Concurrent
d. Skilled

123. Which of the following statements is/ are FALSE about the Risk Adjustment & the Affordable Care Act (ACA)?

a. Calls for a risk adjustment program that aims to eliminate incentives for health insurance plans to avoid people with pre-existing conditions or those who are in poor health.

b. Ensures adjustment that health insurance plans have additional money to provide services to the people who need the most by providing more funds to plans with likely high heath cost.

c. Are added together to recognize the highest paid provider.

d. A and B

124. Which risk adjustment model is used by Medicaid?

a. HCC
b. CDPS
c. Fee for Service
d. Blended

125. Risk adjustment

a. Uses diagnostic information from a base year to predict Medicare benefit costs for the following year
b. Created by CMS
c. Is prospective payment model
d. All the above

126. What does the abbreviation RAPS stand for?

a. Risk Auditing Process System
b. Risk Adjustment Provider Service
c. Risk Adjustment Processing System
d. Risk Auditing Provider System

Quality Care - 6 Questions

127. What does HEDIS stand for?

a. Healthcare, Data Insurance Software
b. Health Effective Data Sets
c. Health Effectiveness Data Information Sets
d. Health Efficient Deal System

128. HEDIS measures are captured by Medicare and Medicaid payers only. HEDIS makes it possible to compare the performance of health plans.

a. True
b. False

129. The purpose of predictive modeling is to anticipate potential future diagnosis for an individual patient.

a. True
b. False

130. To receive a QBP Quality Bonus Payment Medicare advantage plans must be:

a. 3.5 Stars
b. 4.0 Stars
c. 2.5 Stars
d. 3.0 Stars

131. To participate, individual Eps may choose to report quality information though which of the following methods?

a. Qualified PQRS registry
b. Qualified Clinical Data Registry (QCDR)
c. Medicare Part B Claims
d. All the above

132. What are the five domains of care for the 81 HEDIS?

a. Effectiveness of Care, Access and Availability of Care, Experience of Care, Utilization and Relative Resource Use, and Health Plan Descriptive Information.

b. Access and Availability of Care, Experience of Care, Channeling, Utilization, Relative Resource Use, and Health Plan Descriptive Information.

c. Effectiveness of Care, Access and Availability of Care, Experience of Care, Documentation, and Surveys.

d. Access and Availability of Care, Experience of Care, Channeling, Utilization, Relative Resource Use, and Documentation.

Risk Adjustment Models - 18 Questions

133. The CMS-HCC model is a combination of demographic and disease-based factors: What are the demographic variables:

a. Age, Sex, Status, and Medicaid Eligibility
b. Age, Disabled status, Reason for Entitlement, Medicaid Eligibility, and Sex
c. Disabled Status
d. Both A and C are correct

134. Patient presents with COPD and Pulmonary Fibrosis. Using the table below which category should be coded?

CMS-HCC DISEASE HIERARCHIES

If the Disease Group is Listed in This Column...		...Then Drop the Associated Disease Group(s) Listed in This Column	
HCC Disease group	Label	HCC Disease group	Label
112	COPD	111	Pulmonary Fibrosis
110	Cystic Fibrosis	112 111	COPD Pulmonary Fibrosis

a. 112
b. 110
c. 111
d. Both A and B

135. Patient presents with COPD/ Asthma, Pulmonary Fibrosis and Cystic Fibrosis, which HCC should be coded?

a. 110
b. 112
c. Both A and B are correct
d. None of the above are correct

136. Use the table provided below to answer the question.
If the patient is diagnosed with Acute Renal Failure and Dialysis Status, which HCC is used?

If the HCC label is listed in this column...		...Then drop the HCC(s) listed in this column
Hierarchical Condition Category (HCC) Label		
134	Dialysis Status	135,136, 137
135	Acute Renal Failure	136, 137
136	Chronic Kidney Disease, stage 5	137

a. HCC 134 and HCC 135
b. HCC 134
c. HCC 135
d. HCC 136 and HCC 134

137. Which are examples of risked adjustment prescription based programs:

a. MedicaidRx (UCSD)
b. RxGroups (DxCG)
c. Medicare Hierarchical Condition Category, Part D (HCC-D)
d. Health and Human Services Hierarchical Condition Category (HHS HCC-D)
e. All of the above

138. What are the health data elements that accounts for Risk Adjustment?

a. Age, Gender, Socioeconomic status, Years
b. Socioeconomic status, Age, Gender, Disability Status, Claims
c. Disability Status, Medicaid, Age, Gender
d. Medicaid, Age, Gender, Claims

139. Risk Adjustment models are used to evaluate all patients on an equal scale.

a. True
b. False

140. When determining patients-level risk for all risk adjustment models what is used?

a. ICD-10/ ICD9
b. CPT codes
c. HCPCS
d. E & M codes

141. Smoking is a risk factor of:

a. COPD
b. Smokers cough
d. Diabetes
d. Both A and B

142. Internal risk adjustment programs were established to _____.

a. Monitor patient's populations
b. Improve quality care
c. Increase provider engagement
d. All the above are correct

143. What are three main types of reviews for risk adjustment programs?

a. Retroactive, Retrospective, and Concurrent
b. Retrospective, Concurrent, and Prospective
c. Skilled, Concurrent, and Prospective
d. Concurrent, Retroactive, and Prospective

144. An insurance plan comes in to do a risk adjustment review after the data has been reported. What type of chart review is this?

a. Skilled
b. Retrospective
c. Concurrent
d. Prospective

145. Frequency of elements would take visits into consideration for risk adjustments.

a. True
b. False

146. Patient with chronic respiratory failure (84) over rules respiratory arrest (83).

a. True
b. False

147. Tracheostomy status over rules respiratory arrest.

a. True
b. False

148. Patient with history ESRD and chronic respiratory failure was admitted to hospital with respiratory arrest. Patient was unable to breathe on arrival. Patient was intubated and transferred to ICU. Patient is unable to breath on their own, so a temporary trachea was placed. Which is true based off HCC model above?

a. Report ESRD (134) and Tracheostomy Status (82)
b. Chronic Kidney Disease over rule Respiratory Arrest
c. Both A and B
d. Report Respiratory Arrest (84), Tracheostomy Status (82) and ESRD(134)

149. Diabetes reported alone without complications over rules diabetes with complications.

a. True
b. False

150. Which are acceptable for risk adjustment data collection?

a. Hospital Inpatient
b. Hospital Outpatient
c. Physician Services
d. All of the above are correct

Mock Exam - Answers

Compliance - 24 Answers

1. c. Recoup improper payments under Medicare Part C. Medicare Advantage Risk Adjustment Data Validation (RADV) audits are HHS's primary corrective action to recoup improper payments under Medicare Part C.

2. c. Internist.

3. a. True.

4. b. Tabular List and Alphabetic Index.

5. b. False. The classification presumes a causal relationship between the two conditions linked by these terms in the Alphabetic Index or Tabular List. These conditions should be coded as related even in the absence of provider documentation explicitly linking them, unless the documentation clearly states the conditions are unrelated. For conditions not specifically linked by these relational terms in the classification, provider documentation must link the conditions in order to code them as related.

6. a. Deleting the submitted diagnosis codes.

7. b. The definition of fraud and abuse is to purposely bill for services that were never given or to bill for service that has a higher reimbursement than the service provided.

8. d. Both B and C are correct. A compliance plan may offer several benefits, among them – more accurate payments of claims, fewer billing mistakes, improved documentation and more accurate coding, and less chance of violating self- referral and anti-kickback statues.

9. b. Base. By risk adjusting plan bids, CMS can use standardized bids as base payments to plans.

10. a. CMS Medicare is a federal health insurance program administered by Centers for Medicare and Medicaid Services.

11. a. Part A=Inpatient hospitals, skilled facilities, hospice and home health, Part B= Physicians services, outpatient care & preventative services, Part C= Combined benefits of Part A and Part B, D= Prescription drug coverage.

12. c. RAPS; The Risk Adjustment Processing System (RAPS) database contains the diagnostic data submitted by Medicare Advantage plans, PACE organizations, and cost plans.

13. b. In/Outpatient Hospitals, Physician. CMS requires Medicare Advantage plans to collect hospital inpatient, hospital outpatient, and physician risk adjustment data and submit the data to CMS at least quarterly for calculation of the risk score for use in the payment calculation and payment reconciliation. Each quarterly submission should represent approximately one-fourth of the data a plan submits during a data collection year.

14. a. History. The pneumonic "MEAT" is used frequently in risk adjustment coding to represent the criteria for capturing a diagnosis code on a particular date of service. For a diagnosis to be coded on a given date of service, the documentation must clearly state that the specific diagnosis was either Monitored, Evaluated, Assessed or Treated during the face-to-face encounter on that day. Examples of unacceptable documentation sources for risk adjustment coding/ reporting include: Super bills, referral forms, encounter forms, patient-only reported conditions, non face-to-face encounter notes, the stand alone patient problem list. (compliance)

15. d. None of the above. Radiology reports are not acceptable to code from.

16. b. CMS requires the treating provider to sign the medical record in a timely matter within 60 days after the encounter max. Any changes made beyond this time is difficult to justify, and it is unreasonable to assume provider could recall specific details about the encounter.

17. c. CMS. The RADV audits are conducted by CMS to verify the accuracy of the diagnosis codes submitted for payment by the Medicare advantage organization.

18. c. All diagnosis codes reported are supported in the medical record.

19. d. All of the above are correct. In an HRADV (Commercial Risk Adjustment Data Validation), there is an IVA that reviews the sample to identify DOS that supports (through diagnosis codes) for the chosen patients in the sample. IVA is handled by a third-party vendor chosen by the health plan who has no conflicts of interest and can provide both a coding review and the enrollment verification portions of the audit.

20. d. Both A and B. Target RADV audits- target contract of those who have had problematic audits in the past and who have higher risk scores when compared to fee for service Medicare.

21. d. CMS RADV typically involves approximately 45 health plans is NOT true. CMS RADV typically involves approximately 30 health plans.

22. a. ASO. The ASO is the concept is a response to FFS payment.

23. a. Patient/ Caregiver Experience, Care Coordination/ Patient Safety, Preventative Health, At-Risk Population is the correct answer. Heart Failure, Diabetes Measures, and Hypertension Measures are all sub-domain measures, not key domains.

24. a. Code the lowest stage. When provider documentation is between stages such as stage I, II or III, the coder should always choose the lower of the two stages.

Diagnosis Coding - 63 Answers

25. d. E11.65, Z79.4, Z91.128. Patient has uncontrolled diabetes type 2 (E11.65) Insulin Dependent (Z79.4) Patient refuses to take meds (Z91.128)

26. c. S31.000A, B20. Unspecified open wound of lower back and pelvis without penetration into retroperitoneum, initial encounter (S31.000A). Human immunodeficiency virus [HIV] disease (B20).

27. b. I69.354, M06.032, G40.409, I10, E53.8, G63, Z68.41 When coding neuropathy due to other diseases you must code the underlying condition first.

28. a. I82.409, Z79.01. Code acute DVT first and because patient is on anticoagulant use the Z79.01.

29. c. I25.119, Z95.1. Patient has ASHD w/ confirmed angina and s/p CABG stent.

30. d. L89.320 Pressure ulcer of left buttock, unstageable.

31. b. E11.69, E11.22, E11.42.

32. b. R65.20, N17.9, J96.00.

33. d. I12.9, N18.4.

34. d. All the above. International Classification of Diseases -10th Edition - Clinical Modification (ICD-10-CM) Codes 3 to 7 digit codes used to describe the clinical reason for a patient's treatment. The codes do not describe the service performed, just the patient's medical condition. Diagnosis codes drive the risk scores, which drive the risk adjusted reimbursement from CMS to MA organizations. ICD-10-CM codes are used for inpatient discharges on and after the implementation date of ICD-10, and for outpatient and physician services on and after that date.

35. b. I16.1. Hypertensive emergency.

36. a. G43.119, R53.83. Search for migraine then link the aura.

37. d. All the above are correct. A late effect may occur immediately, or months or years later.

38. d. Both A and B are correct. When coding for sequela(e), there are typically two codes that are required. First listed is the condition or nature of the sequela(e); and second, the sequela(e) (late effect).

39. b. E78.5, I10. Hyperlipidemia unspecified is E78.5 and essential hypertension I10.

40. a. I11.0, I50.32. Heart failure preserved ejection failure is Diastolic Heart Failure I50.30 and HFpEf causing Hypertension I11.0.

41. c. I13.2, N18.5, I50.22. Code HTN w/ CKD first then code the type of heart failure.

42. b. Category I83. In ICD-10-CM, the codes for varicose veins are found in category of I83.

43. d. All of the above are correct. ICD-10-CM equates pressure ulcers to bed sores, decubitus and plastic ulcers, pressure ulcers, pressure area or pressure sores.

44. c. Six characters. In ICD10-CM, all pressure ulcers are (L89.-) requires six characters.

45. b. M80.021D. Age-related Osteoporosis with current pathological fracture, right humerus, subsequent encounter for fracture with routine healing.

46. d. N18.6, N25.81, Z99.2. When CKD and ESRD are documented for the same patient, at the same visit, report only ESRD. When reporting ESRD, an additional code should be reported to identify dialysis.

47. a. True. A Patient who undergoes a kidney transplant may continue to have Chronic Kidney Disease because kidneys are not restored to their full function.

48. c. L89.329, L89.319. When multiple sites are documented, select a code for each anatomic site and stage. The sequence depends on the pressure ulcer being treated, sequence the more one severe first.

49. c. L89.623, L89.222. The sequence depends on the pressure ulcer being treated, sequence the more severe first.

50. c. L03.317. Cellulitis of buttock.

51. b.12th Chapter.

52. d. All of the above are correct. Chapter 12 classifies disease and disorders of the nails, hair, hair follicles, sweat glands, sebaceous glands, epidermis, dermis, and subcutaneous tissue.

53. a. 134.

54. d. All of the above. 2016/17 Medicare HCC Categories are infections, blood, neoplasms, substance abuse, metabolic, vascular, liver, openings, amputations, kidney and many more.

55. b. K29.70; Coders should not report signs and symptoms if diagnosed with effect of the symptoms.

56. d. C34.90, C78.7. Primary lung cancer is C34.90 and C78.7 is Secondary (mets) liver.

57. b. E66.01. Morbid obesity code E66.01 should not have been reported because patient is obese E66.9.

58. c. M46.1, J44.9, E11.9, G63, E53.9, J41, Z79.4, G56.00: M46.1 Sacroiliitis J44.9 COPD, E11.9 Diabetes, G63 Vitamin B in neuropathy, E53.9 Vitamin B deficiency, J41 Smokers cough, Z79.4 Insulin Dependent, G56.00. ICD-10 codes should only be reported if there is enough support/ MEAT or if it is a chronic condition.

59. c. Both A and C are correct. If in the assessment section of an EMR states Diabetes – E11.9 then E11.9 should be coded because Diabetes without complications is E11.9. In the assessment section of an EMR record states HTN (I12.9), Smokers cough (J41), ESRD (N18.6), then I12.9, N18.6, J41 should be coded. F33.41 is major depression in partial remission, provider only stated Major depression which is F32.9. E11.43 is not the correct ICD-10-CM for Diabetes with neuropathy.

60. d. F33.0 is the appropriate code for major depression recurrent mild.

61. a. C79.62 is the appropriate code. Secondary malignant neoplasm to the left ovary.

62. c. E70.319, G63. When coding neuropathy in other diseases you must first code the underlying condition in which this case it is E70.319 Albinism and G63 polyneuropathy in other diseases follow.

63. a. D07.1 is the correct code for carcinoma in situ of vulva.

64. b. Z87.891 is the correct code because patient is a current smoker.

65. a. S90.32XA, W55.19XA, Y93.K3 are the correct codes. One activity code from category Y93 is assigned at the initial encounter only to describe the activity of the patient at the time the injury occurred.

66. d. D14.1 is the correct code for benign neoplasm of the larynx.

67. d. E44.0. Moderate protein calorie malnutrition.

68. c. I63.9, I69.954. Per ICD-10-CM guideline I.C.7.d.2, tells us codes from category I69 may be assigned on a health care record with codes from I60-I67, if the patient has a current CVA and deficits from an old CVA. Look in the ICD-10-CM Alphabetic Index for Accident/cerebrovascular (current) I63.9. Also look for Sequela (of)/ disease/cerebrovascular/hemiplegia I69.95-. ICD-10-CM guideline I.C.6.a indicates: Should the affected side be documented, but not specified as dominant or non-dominant, and the classification system does not indicate a default, code selection is as follows: For ambidextrous patients, the default should be dominant; If the left side is affected, the default is non-dominant; if the right side is affected, the default is dominant.

69. d. I48.91, I11.9, I43. Per ICD-10-CM guideline I.C.9.a. indicates: The classification presumes a causal relationship between hypertension and heart involvement, as two conditions are linked by the term "with" in the Alphabetic Index. These conditions should be coded as related even in the absence of provider documentation explicitly linking them, unless the documentation clearly states the conditions are unrelated.

70. d. E11.65, M86.171, Z79.4. Type 2 diabetes mellitus with hyperglycemia is E11.65. Other acute osteomyelitis, right ankle and foot is M86.171. Long term (current) use of insulin is Z79.4. M86.172 was used as diversion as it is of the left foot.

71. c. E89.2. The only risk code in this note is parathyroidectomy.

72. b. G80.9, G23.8, E23.6. These are the only codes mapped for risk purposes.

73. d. G62.0, T40.2X5D. When coding drug induced neuropathy if applicable you must add the secondary code.

74. b. I21.3. Myocardial infarction can be coded while it is equal to, less than, four weeks old.

75. d. Both A and B are correct. Brackets [ ] are used in the tabular list to enclose synonyms, alternate wordings, or explanatory phrases.

76. b. D57.1. Sickle-cell/Hb-C disease without crisis.

77. d. M48.46XS. To report codes M48.4 accurately, a 7th character extender is required. Because the codes themselves are only five characters long, the placeholder X must be used for the 6th character so the 7th character stays in the 7th character position.

78. a. C50.921. Malignant neoplasm of unspecified site of right male breast.

79. d. All of the above. The 4th character in an ICD-10-CM code further defines: The site, etiology, and manifestations or state of disease/ conditions.

80. a. A78, I39. The code first note indicates the codes listed should be sequenced first. If a patient developed endocarditis due to Q fever, the proper codes and sequencing are A78 and I39 for endocarditis.

81. d. I27.82, Z79.01. In the notes for Chronic pulmonary embolism (I27.82) it instructs you to "Use additional code, if applicable, for associated long-term (current) use of anticoagulants (Z79.01).

82. d. M25.511, M25.512. Pain in right shoulder is M25.511, Pain in left shoulder is M25.512.

83. d. All of the above. The correct code for COPD can be found by looking under: Obstruction/ lung/ disease/ chronic, Disease/ lung/ obstruction, Disease/ pulmonary / chronic obstruction.

84. b. Certain. In the outpatient setting, DO NOT CODE a diagnosis unless it is certain. Examples of languages seen in the medical record that identify uncertain diagnoses include Probable, Suspected, Suggestive, Maybe, Rule out, Working, or Differential.

85. a. R53.83. When a definitive diagnosis has not been identified, code signs and symptoms and abnormal testing or other reason for visit.

86. d. K35.80. Coder should not report signs and symptoms with a confirmed diagnosis if the signs or symptom are integral to the diagnosis. For example, the patient is experiencing chest pain, abdominal pain, nauseas and vomiting and the diagnosis is Acute Appendicitis. A symptom code is used with a confirmed diagnosis only when the symptom is not associated with that confirmed diagnosis. It's the coder's responsibility to understand pathophysiology (or to query the provider), to determine if the signs/symptoms may be separately reported or if they are integral to a definitive diagnosis already reported.

87. d. Both B and C are correct. R53.82, R04.2, A15.9. In the hospital/ inpatient setting it is appropriate to report suspected or rule out diagnoses as if the condition does exist. This is only true for facility reporting for inpatient services for all diagnosis except for HIV. HIV is the only condition that must be confirmed if it is to be reported in the inpatient setting.

Documentation Improvement - 18 Answers

88. d. Recommend providers to update history of Prostate cancer to Active Prostate Cancer because patient is on treatment. The cancer is active and there is ongoing treatment with Lupron.

89. c. Coding is the process of translating this written or dictated medical record into a series of numeric or alpha-numeric codes.

90. d. A/P Mild CKD.

91. d. Chronic Bronchitis.

92. d. Risk factors are noted elements about a patient known medical history or social habits that may place the patient at risk for to develop a condition.

93. a. Helps identify those patients who may have a higher medical need than others.

94. d. Recommend confirming the correct site of sciatica. Before coding be sure to read the progress note accurately. The chief complaint is contraindicating.

95. a. True. Medical documentation reviews are used to forecast future health needs, while explaining current needs and expenses.

96. b. Providers signatures and credentials. Providers signatures and credentials are the utmost importance in all documentation efforts.

97. b. "finalized by" is an acceptable signature. Any electronic signature/ authenticated.

98. c. Reporting the diagnosis code alone is not appropriate documentation.

99. d. Both A and C are correct. The Official Guidelines for Coding and Reporting for Outpatient Services, state, "Chronic diseases treated on an ongoing basis may be coded and reported as many times as the patient receives treatment and care for the conditions(s). "Code all documented conditions that coexist at the time of the encounter/visit and require or affect patient care treatment or management. Do not code conditions that were previously treated and no longer exist." This information was previously published in Coding Clinic, Fourth Quarter 2006, pages 236-240.

CMS RAPS Participant Manual: Co-existing conditions include chronic, ongoing conditions such as diabetes (250.XX, HCCs 15-19), congestive heart failure (428.0, HCC 80), atrial fibrillation (427.31, HCC 92), chronic obstructive and pulmonary disease (496, HCC 108). These diseases are generally managed by ongoing medication and have the potential for acute exacerbations if not treated properly, particularly if the patient is experiencing other acute conditions. It is likely that these diagnoses would be part of a general overview of the patient's health when treating co-existing conditions for all but the most minor of medical encounters.

Co-existing conditions also include ongoing conditions such as multiple sclerosis (340, HCC 72), hemiplegia (342.9X, HCC 100), rheumatoid arthritis (714.0, HCC 38) and Parkinson's disease (332.0, HCC 73). Although they may not impact every minor healthcare episode, it is likely that patients having these conditions would have their general health status evaluated within a data reporting period, and these diagnoses would be documented and reportable at that time.

100. d. Diabetes manifestation and the ulcer of the left greater toe. Per ICD-10-CM guideline casual and most common manifestations are ulcers.

101. a. History of DVT, no longer on coumadin. Patient is no longer on treatment so it is appropriate to assign history code.

102. c. Radiology reports. Radiology services are non-covered facilities and should not be used for data collection unless reviewed, signed and documented on Providers Outpatient note.

103. d. Both A and B are correct. Hypertension may have a cause and effect relationship that may lead to a different condition selection. The classification presumes a causal relationship between hypertension and heart involvement and hypertension and kidney involvement. These can be coded in absence of provider documentation.

104. d. A and C. Arrows use of up and down are unacceptable. Coders should not report a diagnosis based on an arrow. HIV should never be reported unless confirmed.

105. d. All of the above. Providers must understand how risk adjustment models work and the models' purposes, the reporting of all diagnosis is important to establish the right risk adjustment factors and HRADV is conducted annually.

Pathophysiology/ Medical Terminology/ Anatomy - 9 Answers

106. a. Filter the blood to remove waste and produce urine. The top 5 functions of your kidneys are remove waste and produce urine, control blood pressure, make red blood cells, control PH levels and keep bones healthy.

107. d. Both B and C are correct. COPD is a group of diseases that affect your lungs and your ability to breathe. The disease blocks the flow of oxygen from your lungs to your blood. This also prevents oxygen from reaching the rest of your body. COPD is primarily caused by smoking and the damage to your lungs can't be reversed.

108. a. Alveoli. Emphysema is a disease of the alveoli. The fibers that make up the walls of the alveoli become damaged. The damage makes them less elastic and unable to work when you exhale.

109. b. Thoracic Cavity; Provide oxygen and nutrients to body tissues by transporting the blood throughout the body. The heart is a muscular organ about the size of a closed fist that functions as the body's circulatory pump. It takes in deoxygenated blood through the veins and delivers it to the lungs for oxygenation before pumping it into the various arteries (which provide oxygen and nutrients to body tissues by transporting the blood throughout the body). The heart is in the thoracic cavity medial to the lungs and posterior to the sternum.

110. b. Respiratory.

111. c. Three. The heart is composed of three layers: epicardium, myocardium, and endocardium.

112. a. Cardi/o, my/o, pathy. The word "cardiomyopathy can be broken down to cardio- heart, myo- muscle, pathy – disease.

113. c. The nervous system is comprised of two parts (central nervous system (brain and spinal cord) and Peripheral nervous system (nerves).

114. a. The muscle surrounding the left ventricle is stronger and larger that of the right ventricle, because the left side is responsible for pumping the blood throughout the entire body.

Purpose and Use of Risk Adjustment Models - 12 Answers

115. a. To allow CMS to pay plans for the risk of the beneficiaries they enroll. By risk adjusting plan payments, CMS can make appropriate and accurate payments for enrollees with differences in expected costs. Increased accuracy benefits patients, providers, health plans, and the nation as a whole.

116. b. Every 12 months. Chronic and acute condition/ diagnoses from the previous year that risk adjust are used to establish reimbursement for patient care provided by Medicare plan. HCCs must be captured every 12 months for CMS reimbursement.

117. d. All of the answers are correct. The following are the segments of the ESRD model: Dialysis, Transplant, and Post-Graft/ Functioning Graft.

118. b. False. Qualified physician data for risk adjustment requires a face-to-face visit except for pathology services (professional component only).

119. d. Future Models. Valid diagnosis codes are those that are published for the fiscal years pertaining to the CMS-HCC risk adjustment model in use for a particular payment year. Current model diagnosis codes are codes that CMS accepts as valid, and are also included in the current version of the CMS-HCC model. Only these diagnosis codes affect the risk score in a payment year. Future model diagnosis codes are codes that are currently valid, but are not included in the current version of the CMS-HCC model and, therefore, do not count toward the risk score.

120. a. Not all ICD codes carry value in risk adjustment models.

121. b. Prospective. Reviews that will affect the next year and not the current year are called Prospective Reviews.

122. c. Concurrent.

123. c. Are added together to recognize the highest paid provider is false. The Affordable Care Act calls for a risk adjustment program that aims to eliminate incentives for health insurance plans to avoid people with pre-existing conditions or those who are in poor health. Risk adjustment ensures that health insurance plans have additional money to provide services to the people who need them most by providing more funds to plans that provide care to people that are likely to have high health costs. Insurance plans then compete based on quality and service, not based on whether they can sign and retain healthy people" (Larsen, 2011)

124. b. CDPS. The Chronic Illness and Disability Payment System (CDPS) is a diagnostic classification system that Medicaid programs can use to make health-based capitated payments for TANF and disabled Medicaid beneficiaries.

125. d. All of the above. Risk adjustment is a prospective payment model created by CMS. It uses diagnostic information from a base year to predict Medicare benefit costs for the following year.

126. c. Risk Adjustment Processing System.

Quality Care - 6 Answers

127. c. Health Effectiveness Data Information Sets.

128. b. False. There are some HEDIS measures captured by Medicare, Medicaid, and private payers. HEDIS makes it possible to compare the performance of health plans.

129. a. True. Health plans and other health specialist often use predictive modeling to anticipate potential future diagnosis for an individual.

130. b. 4.0 stars. Medicare advantage plans that earn four or more stars in a five-star quality rating system would receive a bonus payment.

131. d. All of the above. To participate, individual Eps may choose to report quality information through one of the following 1. Medicare Part B claims, 2. Qualified PQRS registry, 3. HER, CEHRT, 4. CEHRT via data submission vendor and 5. Qualified Clinical Data Registry (QCDR).

132. a. Effectiveness of Care, Access and Availability of Care, Experience of Care, Utilization and Relative Resource Use, and Health Plan Descriptive Information.

Risk Adjustment Models - 18 Answers

133. b. The CMS-HCC model demographic variables include:

• Age as of February 1st of the payment year.
• Sex of the beneficiary.
• Disabled Status results in the inclusion of additional factors in the risk scores of community residents who are disabled beneficiaries under 65 years old.
  • Original Reason for Entitlement results in the inclusion of a factor in the risk score for beneficiaries 65 years of age or older who were originally entitled to Medicare due to disability; the factor differs by the age and sex of the beneficiary.
  • Medicaid Eligibility results in the inclusion of an additional factor in the risk score. (risk adjustment model)

134. c. 111.

135. a. 110.

136. b. HCC 134. If HCC 134 then it drops HCC 136.

137. e. Prescription based program risk adjustment examples are UCSD, DxCG, HCC-D, HHS- HCC- D.

138. b. Socioeconomic status, Age, Gender, Disability Status, Claims. Risk adjustment is a modern methodology that accounts for known and discovered health data elements, and levels comparisons of wellness among patients. Elements are age, gender, socioeconomic status, disability status, insurance status, claims data and special patient specific conditions.

139. a. True. Cost can vary greatly from one patient to another. Therefor risk adjustment models are used to evaluate all patients on an equal scale.

140. a. ICD-10/ ICD-9. All risk adjustment models use diagnosis codes to determine potential patient level risks.

141. d. Both A and B. Smoking can be a risk factor to many different conditions, however, the most common are COPD and Smokers cough.

142. d. All the above are correct. Health plans and risk bearing provider groups establish internal risk adjustment programs to help monitor the patient population, improve quality care, increase provider engagement, and increase accuracy and completeness of data submission to achieve more accurate RAF scores.

143. b. The three main types of reviews are retrospective, concurrent, and prospective.

144. b. Retrospective.

145. b. False. Frequency of elements would NOT take visits into consideration for risk adjustments because patients should be seen by a provider face to face at least once. Frequency visits are not necessary.

146. b. False. Chronic respiratory failure does not over rule respiratory arrest. Based on HCC Model if a patient has respiratory arrest then HCC category 84 must drop off.

147. a. True. Tracheostomy status over rules respiratory arrest. When diagnosis is listed in HCC82 then HCC group 83 and 84 must drop off.

148. a. Report ESRD (134) and Tracheostomy Status (82), based on HCC Model if patient has Respiratory Arrest (83) then (84) Chronic Respiratory Failure should be dropped. And ESRD is not related so both HCC groups can be reported for additional credit.

149. b. False. Families or hierarchies set values based on severity of illness with more severe diagnosis carrying overall risk score than family.

150. d. All of the above are correct. Hospital inpatient, hospital outpatient, and physician services are all acceptable data sources for risk adjustment.

Scoring Sheets
Tear out for easy use

1)	A	B	C	D	27)	A	B	C	D	55)	A	B	C	D
2)	A	B	C	D	28)	A	B	C	D	56)	A	B	C	D
3)	A	B	C	D	29)	A	B	C	D	57)	A	B	C	D
4)	A	B	C	D	30)	A	B	C	D	58)	A	B	C	D
5)	A	B	C	D	31)	A	B	C	D	59)	A	B	C	D
6)	A	B	C	D	32)	A	B	C	D	60)	A	B	C	D
7)	A	B	C	D	33)	A	B	C	D	61)	A	B	C	D
8)	A	B	C	D	34)	A	B	C	D	62)	A	B	C	D
9)	A	B	C	D	35)	A	B	C	D	63)	A	B	C	D
10)	A	B	C	D	36)	A	B	C	D	64)	A	B	C	D
11)	A	B	C	D	37)	A	B	C	D	65)	A	B	C	D
12)	A	B	C	D	38)	A	B	C	D	66)	A	B	C	D
13)	A	B	C	D	39)	A	B	C	D	67)	A	B	C	D
14)	A	B	C	D	40)	A	B	C	D	68)	A	B	C	D
15)	A	B	C	D	41)	A	B	C	D	69)	A	B	C	D
16)	A	B	C	D	42)	A	B	C	D	70)	A	B	C	D
17)	A	B	C	D	43)	A	B	C	D	71)	A	B	C	D
18)	A	B	C	D	44)	A	B	C	D	72)	A	B	C	D
19)	A	B	C	D	45)	A	B	C	D	73)	A	B	C	D
20)	A	B	C	D	46)	A	B	C	D	74)	A	B	C	D
21)	A	B	C	D	47)	A	B	C	D	75)	A	B	C	D
22)	A	B	C	D	48)	A	B	C	D	76)	A	B	C	D
23)	A	B	C	D	49)	A	B	C	D	77)	A	B	C	D
24)	A	B	C	D	50)	A	B	C	D	78)	A	B	C	D
25)	A	B	C	D	51)	A	B	C	D	79)	A	B	C	D
26)	A	B	C	D	52)	A	B	C	D	80)	A	B	C	D
					53)	A	B	C	D	81)	A	B	C	D
					54)	A	B	C	D	82)	A	B	C	D

83)	A	B	C	D	111)	A	B	C	D	139)	A	B	C	D
84)	A	B	C	D	112)	A	B	C	D	140)	A	B	C	D
85)	A	B	C	D	113)	A	B	C	D	141)	A	B	C	D
86)	A	B	C	D	114)	A	B	C	D	142)	A	B	C	D
87)	A	B	C	D	115)	A	B	C	D	143)	A	B	C	D
88)	A	B	C	D	116)	A	B	C	D	144)	A	B	C	D
89)	A	B	C	D	117)	A	B	C	D	145)	A	B	C	D
90)	A	B	C	D	118)	A	B	C	D	146)	A	B	C	D
91)	A	B	C	D	119)	A	B	C	D	147)	A	B	C	D
92)	A	B	C	D	120)	A	B	C	D	148)	A	B	C	D
93)	A	B	C	D	121)	A	B	C	D	149)	A	B	C	D
94)	A	B	C	D	122)	A	B	C	D	150)	A	B	C	D
95)	A	B	C	D	123)	A	B	C	D					
96)	A	B	C	D	124)	A	B	C	D					
97)	A	B	C	D	125)	A	B	C	D					
98)	A	B	C	D	126)	A	B	C	D					
99)	A	B	C	D	127)	A	B	C	D					
100)	A	B	C	D	128)	A	B	C	D					
101)	A	B	C	D	129)	A	B	C	D					
102)	A	B	C	D	130)	A	B	C	D					
103)	A	B	C	D	131)	A	B	C	D					
104)	A	B	C	D	132)	A	B	C	D					
105)	A	B	C	D	133)	A	B	C	D					
106)	A	B	C	D	134)	A	B	C	D					
107)	A	B	C	D	135)	A	B	C	D					
108)	A	B	C	D	136)	A	B	C	D					
109)	A	B	C	D	137)	A	B	C	D					
110)	A	B	C	D	138)	A	B	C	D					

XXXXXXXXXXXXXX
XXXXXXXXXXXXXX
XXXXXXXXXXXXXX
XXXXXXXXXXXXXX

Scoring Sheet 2
Tear out for easy use

1)	A	B	C	D	27)	A	B	C	D	54)	A	B	C	D
2)	A	B	C	D	28)	A	B	C	D	55)	A	B	C	D
3)	A	B	C	D	29)	A	B	C	D	56)	A	B	C	D
4)	A	B	C	D	30)	A	B	C	D	57)	A	B	C	D
5)	A	B	C	D	31)	A	B	C	D	58)	A	B	C	D
6)	A	B	C	D	32)	A	B	C	D	59)	A	B	C	D
7)	A	B	C	D	33)	A	B	C	D	60)	A	B	C	D
8)	A	B	C	D	34)	A	B	C	D	61)	A	B	C	D
9)	A	B	C	D	35)	A	B	C	D	62)	A	B	C	D
10)	A	B	C	D	36)	A	B	C	D	63)	A	B	C	D
11)	A	B	C	D	37)	A	B	C	D	64)	A	B	C	D
12)	A	B	C	D	38)	A	B	C	D	65)	A	B	C	D
13)	A	B	C	D	39)	A	B	C	D	66)	A	B	C	D
14)	A	B	C	D	40)	A	B	C	D	67)	A	B	C	D
15)	A	B	C	D	41)	A	B	C	D	68)	A	B	C	D
16)	A	B	C	D	42)	A	B	C	D	69)	A	B	C	D
17)	A	B	C	D	43)	A	B	C	D	70)	A	B	C	D
18)	A	B	C	D	44)	A	B	C	D	71)	A	B	C	D
19)	A	B	C	D	45)	A	B	C	D	72)	A	B	C	D
20)	A	B	C	D	46)	A	B	C	D	73)	A	B	C	D
21)	A	B	C	D	47)	A	B	C	D	74)	A	B	C	D
22)	A	B	C	D	48)	A	B	C	D	75)	A	B	C	D
23)	A	B	C	D	49)	A	B	C	D	76)	A	B	C	D
24)	A	B	C	D	50)	A	B	C	D	77)	A	B	C	D
25)	A	B	C	D	51)	A	B	C	D	78)	A	B	C	D
26)	A	B	C	D	52)	A	B	C	D	79)	A	B	C	D
					53)	A	B	C	D	80)	A	B	C	D

81)	A	B	C	D	108)	A	B	C	D	135)	A	B	C	D
82)	A	B	C	D	109)	A	B	C	D	136)	A	B	C	D
83)	A	B	C	D	110)	A	B	C	D	137)	A	B	C	D
84)	A	B	C	D	111)	A	B	C	D	138)	A	B	C	D
85)	A	B	C	D	112)	A	B	C	D	139)	A	B	C	D
86)	A	B	C	D	113)	A	B	C	D	140)	A	B	C	D
87)	A	B	C	D	114)	A	B	C	D	141)	A	B	C	D
88)	A	B	C	D	115)	A	B	C	D	142)	A	B	C	D
89)	A	B	C	D	116)	A	B	C	D	143)	A	B	C	D
90)	A	B	C	D	117)	A	B	C	D	144)	A	B	C	D
91)	A	B	C	D	118)	A	B	C	D	145)	A	B	C	D
92)	A	B	C	D	119)	A	B	C	D	146)	A	B	C	D
93)	A	B	C	D	120)	A	B	C	D	147)	A	B	C	D
94)	A	B	C	D	121)	A	B	C	D	148)	A	B	C	D
95)	A	B	C	D	122)	A	B	C	D	149)	A	B	C	D
96)	A	B	C	D	123)	A	B	C	D	150)	A	B	C	D
97)	A	B	C	D	124)	A	B	C	D					
98)	A	B	C	D	125)	A	B	C	D					
99)	A	B	C	D	126)	A	B	C	D					
100)	A	B	C	D	127)	A	B	C	D					
101)	A	B	C	D	128)	A	B	C	D					
102)	A	B	C	D	129)	A	B	C	D					
103)	A	B	C	D	130)	A	B	C	D					
104)	A	B	C	D	131)	A	B	C	D					
105)	A	B	C	D	132)	A	B	C	D					
106)	A	B	C	D	133)	A	B	C	D					
107)	A	B	C	D	134)	A	B	C	D					

XXXXXXXXXXXXXX
XXXXXXXXXXXXXX
XXXXXXXXXXXXXX
XXXXXXXXXXXXXX

Scoring Sheet 3
Tear out for easy use

1)	A	B	C	D	26)	A	B	C	D	53)	A	B	C	D
2)	A	B	C	D	27)	A	B	C	D	54)	A	B	C	D
3)	A	B	C	D	28)	A	B	C	D	55)	A	B	C	D
4)	A	B	C	D	29)	A	B	C	D	56)	A	B	C	D
5)	A	B	C	D	30)	A	B	C	D	57)	A	B	C	D
6)	A	B	C	D	31)	A	B	C	D	58)	A	B	C	D
7)	A	B	C	D	32)	A	B	C	D	59)	A	B	C	D
8)	A	B	C	D	33)	A	B	C	D	60)	A	B	C	D
9)	A	B	C	D	34)	A	B	C	D	61)	A	B	C	D
10)	A	B	C	D	35)	A	B	C	D	62)	A	B	C	D
11)	A	B	C	D	36)	A	B	C	D	63)	A	B	C	D
12)	A	B	C	D	37)	A	B	C	D	64)	A	B	C	D
13)	A	B	C	D	38)	A	B	C	D	65)	A	B	C	D
14)	A	B	C	D	39)	A	B	C	D	66)	A	B	C	D
15)	A	B	C	D	40)	A	B	C	D	67)	A	B	C	D
16)	A	B	C	D	41)	A	B	C	D	68)	A	B	C	D
17)	A	B	C	D	42)	A	B	C	D	69)	A	B	C	D
18)	A	B	C	D	43)	A	B	C	D	70)	A	B	C	D
19)	A	B	C	D	44)	A	B	C	D	71)	A	B	C	D
20)	A	B	C	D	45)	A	B	C	D	72)	A	B	C	D
21)	A	B	C	D	46)	A	B	C	D	73)	A	B	C	D
22)	A	B	C	D	47)	A	B	C	D	74)	A	B	C	D
23)	A	B	C	D	48)	A	B	C	D	75)	A	B	C	D
24)	A	B	C	D	49)	A	B	C	D	76)	A	B	C	D
25)	A	B	C	D	50)	A	B	C	D	77)	A	B	C	D
					51)	A	B	C	D	78)	A	B	C	D
					52)	A	B	C	D	79)	A	B	C	D

80)	A	B	C	D	107)	A	B	C	D	134)	A	B	C	D
81)	A	B	C	D	108)	A	B	C	D	135)	A	B	C	D
82)	A	B	C	D	109)	A	B	C	D	136)	A	B	C	D
83)	A	B	C	D	110)	A	B	C	D	137)	A	B	C	D
84)	A	B	C	D	111)	A	B	C	D	138)	A	B	C	D
85)	A	B	C	D	112)	A	B	C	D	139)	A	B	C	D
86)	A	B	C	D	113)	A	B	C	D	140)	A	B	C	D
87)	A	B	C	D	114)	A	B	C	D	141)	A	B	C	D
88)	A	B	C	D	115)	A	B	C	D	142)	A	B	C	D
89)	A	B	C	D	116)	A	B	C	D	143)	A	B	C	D
90)	A	B	C	D	117)	A	B	C	D	144)	A	B	C	D
91)	A	B	C	D	118)	A	B	C	D	145)	A	B	C	D
92)	A	B	C	D	119)	A	B	C	D	146)	A	B	C	D
93)	A	B	C	D	120)	A	B	C	D	147)	A	B	C	D
94)	A	B	C	D	121)	A	B	C	D	148)	A	B	C	D
95)	A	B	C	D	122)	A	B	C	D	149)	A	B	C	D
96)	A	B	C	D	123)	A	B	C	D	150)	A	B	C	D
97)	A	B	C	D	124)	A	B	C	D					
98)	A	B	C	D	125)	A	B	C	D					
99)	A	B	C	D	126)	A	B	C	D					
100)	A	B	C	D	127)	A	B	C	D					
101)	A	B	C	D	128)	A	B	C	D					
102)	A	B	C	D	129)	A	B	C	D					
103)	A	B	C	D	130)	A	B	C	D					
104)	A	B	C	D	131)	A	B	C	D					
105)	A	B	C	D	132)	A	B	C	D					
106)	A	B	C	D	133)	A	B	C	D					

XXXXXXXXXXXXXX
XXXXXXXXXXXXXX
XXXXXXXXXXXXXX
XXXXXXXXXXXXXX

Scoring Sheet 4
Tear out for easy use

1)	A	B	C	D	26)	A	B	C	D	53)	A	B	C	D
2)	A	B	C	D	27)	A	B	C	D	54)	A	B	C	D
3)	A	B	C	D	28)	A	B	C	D	55)	A	B	C	D
4)	A	B	C	D	29)	A	B	C	D	56)	A	B	C	D
5)	A	B	C	D	30)	A	B	C	D	57)	A	B	C	D
6)	A	B	C	D	31)	A	B	C	D	58)	A	B	C	D
7)	A	B	C	D	32)	A	B	C	D	59)	A	B	C	D
8)	A	B	C	D	33)	A	B	C	D	60)	A	B	C	D
9)	A	B	C	D	34)	A	B	C	D	61)	A	B	C	D
10)	A	B	C	D	35)	A	B	C	D	62)	A	B	C	D
11)	A	B	C	D	36)	A	B	C	D	63)	A	B	C	D
12)	A	B	C	D	37)	A	B	C	D	64)	A	B	C	D
13)	A	B	C	D	38)	A	B	C	D	65)	A	B	C	D
14)	A	B	C	D	39)	A	B	C	D	66)	A	B	C	D
15)	A	B	C	D	40)	A	B	C	D	67)	A	B	C	D
16)	A	B	C	D	41)	A	B	C	D	68)	A	B	C	D
17)	A	B	C	D	42)	A	B	C	D	69)	A	B	C	D
18)	A	B	C	D	43)	A	B	C	D	70)	A	B	C	D
19)	A	B	C	D	44)	A	B	C	D	71)	A	B	C	D
20)	A	B	C	D	45)	A	B	C	D	72)	A	B	C	D
21)	A	B	C	D	46)	A	B	C	D	73)	A	B	C	D
22)	A	B	C	D	47)	A	B	C	D	74)	A	B	C	D
23)	A	B	C	D	48)	A	B	C	D	75)	A	B	C	D
24)	A	B	C	D	49)	A	B	C	D	76)	A	B	C	D
25)	A	B	C	D	50)	A	B	C	D	77)	A	B	C	D
					51)	A	B	C	D	78)	A	B	C	D
					52)	A	B	C	D	79)	A	B	C	D

80)	A	B	C	D	107)	A	B	C	D	134)	A	B	C	D
81)	A	B	C	D	108)	A	B	C	D	135)	A	B	C	D
82)	A	B	C	D	109)	A	B	C	D	136)	A	B	C	D
83)	A	B	C	D	110)	A	B	C	D	137)	A	B	C	D
84)	A	B	C	D	111)	A	B	C	D	138)	A	B	C	D
85)	A	B	C	D	112)	A	B	C	D	139)	A	B	C	D
86)	A	B	C	D	113)	A	B	C	D	140)	A	B	C	D
87)	A	B	C	D	114)	A	B	C	D	141)	A	B	C	D
88)	A	B	C	D	115)	A	B	C	D	142)	A	B	C	D
89)	A	B	C	D	116)	A	B	C	D	143)	A	B	C	D
90)	A	B	C	D	117)	A	B	C	D	144)	A	B	C	D
91)	A	B	C	D	118)	A	B	C	D	145)	A	B	C	D
92)	A	B	C	D	119)	A	B	C	D	146)	A	B	C	D
93)	A	B	C	D	120)	A	B	C	D	147)	A	B	C	D
94)	A	B	C	D	121)	A	B	C	D	148)	A	B	C	D
95)	A	B	C	D	122)	A	B	C	D	149)	A	B	C	D
96)	A	B	C	D	123)	A	B	C	D	150)	A	B	C	D
97)	A	B	C	D	124)	A	B	C	D					
98)	A	B	C	D	125)	A	B	C	D					
99)	A	B	C	D	126)	A	B	C	D					
100)	A	B	C	D	127)	A	B	C	D					
101)	A	B	C	D	128)	A	B	C	D					
102)	A	B	C	D	129)	A	B	C	D					
103)	A	B	C	D	130)	A	B	C	D					
104)	A	B	C	D	131)	A	B	C	D					
105)	A	B	C	D	132)	A	B	C	D					
106)	A	B	C	D	133)	A	B	C	D					

XXXXXXXXXXXXXX
XXXXXXXXXXXXXX
XXXXXXXXXXXXXX
XXXXXXXXXXXXXX

Scoring Sheet 5
Tear out for easy use

1) A B C D
2) A B C D
3) A B C D
4) A B C D
5) A B C D
6) A B C D
7) A B C D
8) A B C D
9) A B C D
10) A B C D
11) A B C D
12) A B C D
13) A B C D
14) A B C D
15) A B C D
16) A B C D
17) A B C D
18) A B C D
19) A B C D
20) A B C D
21) A B C D
22) A B C D
23) A B C D
24) A B C D
25) A B C D

26) A B C D
27) A B C D
28) A B C D
29) A B C D
30) A B C D
31) A B C D
32) A B C D
33) A B C D
34) A B C D
35) A B C D
36) A B C D
37) A B C D
38) A B C D
39) A B C D
40) A B C D
41) A B C D
42) A B C D
43) A B C D
44) A B C D
45) A B C D
46) A B C D
47) A B C D
48) A B C D
49) A B C D
50) A B C D
51) A B C D
52) A B C D

53) A B C D
54) A B C D
55) A B C D
56) A B C D
57) A B C D
58) A B C D
59) A B C D
60) A B C D
61) A B C D
62) A B C D
63) A B C D
64) A B C D
65) A B C D
66) A B C D
67) A B C D
68) A B C D
69) A B C D
70) A B C D
71) A B C D
72) A B C D
73) A B C D
74) A B C D
75) A B C D
76) A B C D
77) A B C D
78) A B C D
79) A B C D

80)	A	B	C	D	107)	A	B	C	D	134)	A	B	C	D
81)	A	B	C	D	108)	A	B	C	D	135)	A	B	C	D
82)	A	B	C	D	109)	A	B	C	D	136)	A	B	C	D
83)	A	B	C	D	110)	A	B	C	D	137)	A	B	C	D
84)	A	B	C	D	111)	A	B	C	D	138)	A	B	C	D
85)	A	B	C	D	112)	A	B	C	D	139)	A	B	C	D
86)	A	B	C	D	113)	A	B	C	D	140)	A	B	C	D
87)	A	B	C	D	114)	A	B	C	D	141)	A	B	C	D
88)	A	B	C	D	115)	A	B	C	D	142)	A	B	C	D
89)	A	B	C	D	116)	A	B	C	D	143)	A	B	C	D
90)	A	B	C	D	117)	A	B	C	D	144)	A	B	C	D
91)	A	B	C	D	118)	A	B	C	D	145)	A	B	C	D
92)	A	B	C	D	119)	A	B	C	D	146)	A	B	C	D
93)	A	B	C	D	120)	A	B	C	D	147)	A	B	C	D
94)	A	B	C	D	121)	A	B	C	D	148)	A	B	C	D
95)	A	B	C	D	122)	A	B	C	D	149)	A	B	C	D
96)	A	B	C	D	123)	A	B	C	D	150)	A	B	C	D
97)	A	B	C	D	124)	A	B	C	D					
98)	A	B	C	D	125)	A	B	C	D					
99)	A	B	C	D	126)	A	B	C	D					
100)	A	B	C	D	127)	A	B	C	D					
101)	A	B	C	D	128)	A	B	C	D					
102)	A	B	C	D	129)	A	B	C	D					
103)	A	B	C	D	130)	A	B	C	D					
104)	A	B	C	D	131)	A	B	C	D					
105)	A	B	C	D	132)	A	B	C	D					
106)	A	B	C	D	133)	A	B	C	D					

XXXXXXXXXXXXXX
XXXXXXXXXXXXXX
XXXXXXXXXXXXXX
XXXXXXXXXXXXXX

Scoring Sheet 6
Tear out for easy use

1) A B C D
2) A B C D
3) A B C D
4) A B C D
5) A B C D
6) A B C D
7) A B C D
8) A B C D
9) A B C D
10) A B C D
11) A B C D
12) A B C D
13) A B C D
14) A B C D
15) A B C D
16) A B C D
17) A B C D
18) A B C D
19) A B C D
20) A B C D
21) A B C D
22) A B C D
23) A B C D
24) A B C D
25) A B C D

26) A B C D
27) A B C D
28) A B C D
29) A B C D
30) A B C D
31) A B C D
32) A B C D
33) A B C D
34) A B C D
35) A B C D
36) A B C D
37) A B C D
38) A B C D
39) A B C D
40) A B C D
41) A B C D
42) A B C D
43) A B C D
44) A B C D
45) A B C D
46) A B C D
47) A B C D
48) A B C D
49) A B C D
50) A B C D
51) A B C D
52) A B C D

53) A B C D
54) A B C D
55) A B C D
56) A B C D
57) A B C D
58) A B C D
59) A B C D
60) A B C D
61) A B C D
62) A B C D
63) A B C D
64) A B C D
65) A B C D
66) A B C D
67) A B C D
68) A B C D
69) A B C D
70) A B C D
71) A B C D
72) A B C D
73) A B C D
74) A B C D
75) A B C D
76) A B C D
77) A B C D
78) A B C D
79) A B C D

80)	A	B	C	D	107)	A	B	C	D	134)	A	B	C	D
81)	A	B	C	D	108)	A	B	C	D	135)	A	B	C	D
82)	A	B	C	D	109)	A	B	C	D	136)	A	B	C	D
83)	A	B	C	D	110)	A	B	C	D	137)	A	B	C	D
84)	A	B	C	D	111)	A	B	C	D	138)	A	B	C	D
85)	A	B	C	D	112)	A	B	C	D	139)	A	B	C	D
86)	A	B	C	D	113)	A	B	C	D	140)	A	B	C	D
87)	A	B	C	D	114)	A	B	C	D	141)	A	B	C	D
88)	A	B	C	D	115)	A	B	C	D	142)	A	B	C	D
89)	A	B	C	D	116)	A	B	C	D	143)	A	B	C	D
90)	A	B	C	D	117)	A	B	C	D	144)	A	B	C	D
91)	A	B	C	D	118)	A	B	C	D	145)	A	B	C	D
92)	A	B	C	D	119)	A	B	C	D	146)	A	B	C	D
93)	A	B	C	D	120)	A	B	C	D	147)	A	B	C	D
94)	A	B	C	D	121)	A	B	C	D	148)	A	B	C	D
95)	A	B	C	D	122)	A	B	C	D	149)	A	B	C	D
96)	A	B	C	D	123)	A	B	C	D	150)	A	B	C	D
97)	A	B	C	D	124)	A	B	C	D					
98)	A	B	C	D	125)	A	B	C	D					
99)	A	B	C	D	126)	A	B	C	D					
100)	A	B	C	D	127)	A	B	C	D					
101)	A	B	C	D	128)	A	B	C	D					
102)	A	B	C	D	129)	A	B	C	D					
103)	A	B	C	D	130)	A	B	C	D					
104)	A	B	C	D	131)	A	B	C	D					
105)	A	B	C	D	132)	A	B	C	D					
106)	A	B	C	D	133)	A	B	C	D					

XXXXXXXXXXXXXXX
XXXXXXXXXXXXXXX
XXXXXXXXXXXXXXX
XXXXXXXXXXXXXXX

Scoring Sheet 7

Tear out for easy use

1) A B C D
2) A B C D
3) A B C D
4) A B C D
5) A B C D
6) A B C D
7) A B C D
8) A B C D
9) A B C D
10) A B C D
11) A B C D
12) A B C D
13) A B C D
14) A B C D
15) A B C D
16) A B C D
17) A B C D
18) A B C D
19) A B C D
20) A B C D
21) A B C D
22) A B C D
23) A B C D
24) A B C D
25) A B C D

26) A B C D
27) A B C D
28) A B C D
29) A B C D
30) A B C D
31) A B C D
32) A B C D
33) A B C D
34) A B C D
35) A B C D
36) A B C D
37) A B C D
38) A B C D
39) A B C D
40) A B C D
41) A B C D
42) A B C D
43) A B C D
44) A B C D
45) A B C D
46) A B C D
47) A B C D
48) A B C D
49) A B C D
50) A B C D
51) A B C D
52) A B C D

53) A B C D
54) A B C D
55) A B C D
56) A B C D
57) A B C D
58) A B C D
59) A B C D
60) A B C D
61) A B C D
62) A B C D
63) A B C D
64) A B C D
65) A B C D
66) A B C D
67) A B C D
68) A B C D
69) A B C D
70) A B C D
71) A B C D
72) A B C D
73) A B C D
74) A B C D
75) A B C D
76) A B C D
77) A B C D
78) A B C D
79) A B C D

80)	A	B	C	D	107)	A	B	C	D	134)	A	B	C	D
81)	A	B	C	D	108)	A	B	C	D	135)	A	B	C	D
82)	A	B	C	D	109)	A	B	C	D	136)	A	B	C	D
83)	A	B	C	D	110)	A	B	C	D	137)	A	B	C	D
84)	A	B	C	D	111)	A	B	C	D	138)	A	B	C	D
85)	A	B	C	D	112)	A	B	C	D	139)	A	B	C	D
86)	A	B	C	D	113)	A	B	C	D	140)	A	B	C	D
87)	A	B	C	D	114)	A	B	C	D	141)	A	B	C	D
88)	A	B	C	D	115)	A	B	C	D	142)	A	B	C	D
89)	A	B	C	D	116)	A	B	C	D	143)	A	B	C	D
90)	A	B	C	D	117)	A	B	C	D	144)	A	B	C	D
91)	A	B	C	D	118)	A	B	C	D	145)	A	B	C	D
92)	A	B	C	D	119)	A	B	C	D	146)	A	B	C	D
93)	A	B	C	D	120)	A	B	C	D	147)	A	B	C	D
94)	A	B	C	D	121)	A	B	C	D	148)	A	B	C	D
95)	A	B	C	D	122)	A	B	C	D	149)	A	B	C	D
96)	A	B	C	D	123)	A	B	C	D	150)	A	B	C	D
97)	A	B	C	D	124)	A	B	C	D					
98)	A	B	C	D	125)	A	B	C	D					
99)	A	B	C	D	126)	A	B	C	D					
100)	A	B	C	D	127)	A	B	C	D					
101)	A	B	C	D	128)	A	B	C	D					
102)	A	B	C	D	129)	A	B	C	D					
103)	A	B	C	D	130)	A	B	C	D					
104)	A	B	C	D	131)	A	B	C	D					
105)	A	B	C	D	132)	A	B	C	D					
106)	A	B	C	D	133)	A	B	C	D					

XXXXXXXXXXXXXX
XXXXXXXXXXXXXX
XXXXXXXXXXXXXX
XXXXXXXXXXXXXX

Scoring Sheet 8
Tear out for easy use

1)	A	B	C	D	26)	A	B	C	D	53)	A	B	C	D
2)	A	B	C	D	27)	A	B	C	D	54)	A	B	C	D
3)	A	B	C	D	28)	A	B	C	D	55)	A	B	C	D
4)	A	B	C	D	29)	A	B	C	D	56)	A	B	C	D
5)	A	B	C	D	30)	A	B	C	D	57)	A	B	C	D
6)	A	B	C	D	31)	A	B	C	D	58)	A	B	C	D
7)	A	B	C	D	32)	A	B	C	D	59)	A	B	C	D
8)	A	B	C	D	33)	A	B	C	D	60)	A	B	C	D
9)	A	B	C	D	34)	A	B	C	D	61)	A	B	C	D
10)	A	B	C	D	35)	A	B	C	D	62)	A	B	C	D
11)	A	B	C	D	36)	A	B	C	D	63)	A	B	C	D
12)	A	B	C	D	37)	A	B	C	D	64)	A	B	C	D
13)	A	B	C	D	38)	A	B	C	D	65)	A	B	C	D
14)	A	B	C	D	39)	A	B	C	D	66)	A	B	C	D
15)	A	B	C	D	40)	A	B	C	D	67)	A	B	C	D
16)	A	B	C	D	41)	A	B	C	D	68)	A	B	C	D
17)	A	B	C	D	42)	A	B	C	D	69)	A	B	C	D
18)	A	B	C	D	43)	A	B	C	D	70)	A	B	C	D
19)	A	B	C	D	44)	A	B	C	D	71)	A	B	C	D
20)	A	B	C	D	45)	A	B	C	D	72)	A	B	C	D
21)	A	B	C	D	46)	A	B	C	D	73)	A	B	C	D
22)	A	B	C	D	47)	A	B	C	D	74)	A	B	C	D
23)	A	B	C	D	48)	A	B	C	D	75)	A	B	C	D
24)	A	B	C	D	49)	A	B	C	D	76)	A	B	C	D
25)	A	B	C	D	50)	A	B	C	D	77)	A	B	C	D
					51)	A	B	C	D	78)	A	B	C	D
					52)	A	B	C	D	79)	A	B	C	D

80)	A	B	C	D	107)	A	B	C	D	134)	A	B	C	D
81)	A	B	C	D	108)	A	B	C	D	135)	A	B	C	D
82)	A	B	C	D	109)	A	B	C	D	136)	A	B	C	D
83)	A	B	C	D	110)	A	B	C	D	137)	A	B	C	D
84)	A	B	C	D	111)	A	B	C	D	138)	A	B	C	D
85)	A	B	C	D	112)	A	B	C	D	139)	A	B	C	D
86)	A	B	C	D	113)	A	B	C	D	140)	A	B	C	D
87)	A	B	C	D	114)	A	B	C	D	141)	A	B	C	D
88)	A	B	C	D	115)	A	B	C	D	142)	A	B	C	D
89)	A	B	C	D	116)	A	B	C	D	143)	A	B	C	D
90)	A	B	C	D	117)	A	B	C	D	144)	A	B	C	D
91)	A	B	C	D	118)	A	B	C	D	145)	A	B	C	D
92)	A	B	C	D	119)	A	B	C	D	146)	A	B	C	D
93)	A	B	C	D	120)	A	B	C	D	147)	A	B	C	D
94)	A	B	C	D	121)	A	B	C	D	148)	A	B	C	D
95)	A	B	C	D	122)	A	B	C	D	149)	A	B	C	D
96)	A	B	C	D	123)	A	B	C	D	150)	A	B	C	D
97)	A	B	C	D	124)	A	B	C	D					
98)	A	B	C	D	125)	A	B	C	D					
99)	A	B	C	D	126)	A	B	C	D					
100)	A	B	C	D	127)	A	B	C	D					
101)	A	B	C	D	128)	A	B	C	D					
102)	A	B	C	D	129)	A	B	C	D					
103)	A	B	C	D	130)	A	B	C	D					
104)	A	B	C	D	131)	A	B	C	D					
105)	A	B	C	D	132)	A	B	C	D					
106)	A	B	C	D	133)	A	B	C	D					

XXXXXXXXXXXXXX
XXXXXXXXXXXXXX
XXXXXXXXXXXXXX
XXXXXXXXXXXXXX

Scoring Sheet 9
Tear out for easy use

1)	A	B	C	D	26)	A	B	C	D	53)	A	B	C	D
2)	A	B	C	D	27)	A	B	C	D	54)	A	B	C	D
3)	A	B	C	D	28)	A	B	C	D	55)	A	B	C	D
4)	A	B	C	D	29)	A	B	C	D	56)	A	B	C	D
5)	A	B	C	D	30)	A	B	C	D	57)	A	B	C	D
6)	A	B	C	D	31)	A	B	C	D	58)	A	B	C	D
7)	A	B	C	D	32)	A	B	C	D	59)	A	B	C	D
8)	A	B	C	D	33)	A	B	C	D	60)	A	B	C	D
9)	A	B	C	D	34)	A	B	C	D	61)	A	B	C	D
10)	A	B	C	D	35)	A	B	C	D	62)	A	B	C	D
11)	A	B	C	D	36)	A	B	C	D	63)	A	B	C	D
12)	A	B	C	D	37)	A	B	C	D	64)	A	B	C	D
13)	A	B	C	D	38)	A	B	C	D	65)	A	B	C	D
14)	A	B	C	D	39)	A	B	C	D	66)	A	B	C	D
15)	A	B	C	D	40)	A	B	C	D	67)	A	B	C	D
16)	A	B	C	D	41)	A	B	C	D	68)	A	B	C	D
17)	A	B	C	D	42)	A	B	C	D	69)	A	B	C	D
18)	A	B	C	D	43)	A	B	C	D	70)	A	B	C	D
19)	A	B	C	D	44)	A	B	C	D	71)	A	B	C	D
20)	A	B	C	D	45)	A	B	C	D	72)	A	B	C	D
21)	A	B	C	D	46)	A	B	C	D	73)	A	B	C	D
22)	A	B	C	D	47)	A	B	C	D	74)	A	B	C	D
23)	A	B	C	D	48)	A	B	C	D	75)	A	B	C	D
24)	A	B	C	D	49)	A	B	C	D	76)	A	B	C	D
25)	A	B	C	D	50)	A	B	C	D	77)	A	B	C	D
					51)	A	B	C	D	78)	A	B	C	D
					52)	A	B	C	D	79)	A	B	C	D

80)	A	B	C	D	107)	A	B	C	D	134)	A	B	C	D
81)	A	B	C	D	108)	A	B	C	D	135)	A	B	C	D
82)	A	B	C	D	109)	A	B	C	D	136)	A	B	C	D
83)	A	B	C	D	110)	A	B	C	D	137)	A	B	C	D
84)	A	B	C	D	111)	A	B	C	D	138)	A	B	C	D
85)	A	B	C	D	112)	A	B	C	D	139)	A	B	C	D
86)	A	B	C	D	113)	A	B	C	D	140)	A	B	C	D
87)	A	B	C	D	114)	A	B	C	D	141)	A	B	C	D
88)	A	B	C	D	115)	A	B	C	D	142)	A	B	C	D
89)	A	B	C	D	116)	A	B	C	D	143)	A	B	C	D
90)	A	B	C	D	117)	A	B	C	D	144)	A	B	C	D
91)	A	B	C	D	118)	A	B	C	D	145)	A	B	C	D
92)	A	B	C	D	119)	A	B	C	D	146)	A	B	C	D
93)	A	B	C	D	120)	A	B	C	D	147)	A	B	C	D
94)	A	B	C	D	121)	A	B	C	D	148)	A	B	C	D
95)	A	B	C	D	122)	A	B	C	D	149)	A	B	C	D
96)	A	B	C	D	123)	A	B	C	D	150)	A	B	C	D
97)	A	B	C	D	124)	A	B	C	D					
98)	A	B	C	D	125)	A	B	C	D	XXXXXXXXXXXXXXX				
99)	A	B	C	D	126)	A	B	C	D	XXXXXXXXXXXXXXX				
100)	A	B	C	D	127)	A	B	C	D	XXXXXXXXXXXXXXX				
101)	A	B	C	D	128)	A	B	C	D	XXXXXXXXXXXXXXX				
102)	A	B	C	D	129)	A	B	C	D					
103)	A	B	C	D	130)	A	B	C	D					
104)	A	B	C	D	131)	A	B	C	D					
105)	A	B	C	D	132)	A	B	C	D					
106)	A	B	C	D	133)	A	B	C	D					

Scoring Sheet 10
Tear out for easy use

1) A B C D
2) A B C D
3) A B C D
4) A B C D
5) A B C D
6) A B C D
7) A B C D
8) A B C D
9) A B C D
10) A B C D
11) A B C D
12) A B C D
13) A B C D
14) A B C D
15) A B C D
16) A B C D
17) A B C D
18) A B C D
19) A B C D
20) A B C D
21) A B C D
22) A B C D
23) A B C D
24) A B C D
25) A B C D

26) A B C D
27) A B C D
28) A B C D
29) A B C D
30) A B C D
31) A B C D
32) A B C D
33) A B C D
34) A B C D
35) A B C D
36) A B C D
37) A B C D
38) A B C D
39) A B C D
40) A B C D
41) A B C D
42) A B C D
43) A B C D
44) A B C D
45) A B C D
46) A B C D
47) A B C D
48) A B C D
49) A B C D
50) A B C D
51) A B C D
52) A B C D

53) A B C D
54) A B C D
55) A B C D
56) A B C D
57) A B C D
58) A B C D
59) A B C D
60) A B C D
61) A B C D
62) A B C D
63) A B C D
64) A B C D
65) A B C D
66) A B C D
67) A B C D
68) A B C D
69) A B C D
70) A B C D
71) A B C D
72) A B C D
73) A B C D
74) A B C D
75) A B C D
76) A B C D
77) A B C D
78) A B C D
79) A B C D

80)	A	B	C	D	107)	A	B	C	D	134)	A	B	C	D
81)	A	B	C	D	108)	A	B	C	D	135)	A	B	C	D
82)	A	B	C	D	109)	A	B	C	D	136)	A	B	C	D
83)	A	B	C	D	110)	A	B	C	D	137)	A	B	C	D
84)	A	B	C	D	111)	A	B	C	D	138)	A	B	C	D
85)	A	B	C	D	112)	A	B	C	D	139)	A	B	C	D
86)	A	B	C	D	113)	A	B	C	D	140)	A	B	C	D
87)	A	B	C	D	114)	A	B	C	D	141)	A	B	C	D
88)	A	B	C	D	115)	A	B	C	D	142)	A	B	C	D
89)	A	B	C	D	116)	A	B	C	D	143)	A	B	C	D
90)	A	B	C	D	117)	A	B	C	D	144)	A	B	C	D
91)	A	B	C	D	118)	A	B	C	D	145)	A	B	C	D
92)	A	B	C	D	119)	A	B	C	D	146)	A	B	C	D
93)	A	B	C	D	120)	A	B	C	D	147)	A	B	C	D
94)	A	B	C	D	121)	A	B	C	D	148)	A	B	C	D
95)	A	B	C	D	122)	A	B	C	D	149)	A	B	C	D
96)	A	B	C	D	123)	A	B	C	D	150)	A	B	C	D
97)	A	B	C	D	124)	A	B	C	D					
98)	A	B	C	D	125)	A	B	C	D					
99)	A	B	C	D	126)	A	B	C	D					
100)	A	B	C	D	127)	A	B	C	D					
101)	A	B	C	D	128)	A	B	C	D					
102)	A	B	C	D	129)	A	B	C	D					
103)	A	B	C	D	130)	A	B	C	D					
104)	A	B	C	D	131)	A	B	C	D					
105)	A	B	C	D	132)	A	B	C	D					
106)	A	B	C	D	133)	A	B	C	D					

XXXXXXXXXXXXXX
XXXXXXXXXXXXXX
XXXXXXXXXXXXXX
XXXXXXXXXXXXXX

Scoring Sheet 11
Tear out for easy use

1)	A	B	C	D	26)	A	B	C	D	53)	A	B	C	D
2)	A	B	C	D	27)	A	B	C	D	54)	A	B	C	D
3)	A	B	C	D	28)	A	B	C	D	55)	A	B	C	D
4)	A	B	C	D	29)	A	B	C	D	56)	A	B	C	D
5)	A	B	C	D	30)	A	B	C	D	57)	A	B	C	D
6)	A	B	C	D	31)	A	B	C	D	58)	A	B	C	D
7)	A	B	C	D	32)	A	B	C	D	59)	A	B	C	D
8)	A	B	C	D	33)	A	B	C	D	60)	A	B	C	D
9)	A	B	C	D	34)	A	B	C	D	61)	A	B	C	D
10)	A	B	C	D	35)	A	B	C	D	62)	A	B	C	D
11)	A	B	C	D	36)	A	B	C	D	63)	A	B	C	D
12)	A	B	C	D	37)	A	B	C	D	64)	A	B	C	D
13)	A	B	C	D	38)	A	B	C	D	65)	A	B	C	D
14)	A	B	C	D	39)	A	B	C	D	66)	A	B	C	D
15)	A	B	C	D	40)	A	B	C	D	67)	A	B	C	D
16)	A	B	C	D	41)	A	B	C	D	68)	A	B	C	D
17)	A	B	C	D	42)	A	B	C	D	69)	A	B	C	D
18)	A	B	C	D	43)	A	B	C	D	70)	A	B	C	D
19)	A	B	C	D	44)	A	B	C	D	71)	A	B	C	D
20)	A	B	C	D	45)	A	B	C	D	72)	A	B	C	D
21)	A	B	C	D	46)	A	B	C	D	73)	A	B	C	D
22)	A	B	C	D	47)	A	B	C	D	74)	A	B	C	D
23)	A	B	C	D	48)	A	B	C	D	75)	A	B	C	D
24)	A	B	C	D	49)	A	B	C	D	76)	A	B	C	D
25)	A	B	C	D	50)	A	B	C	D	77)	A	B	C	D
					51)	A	B	C	D	78)	A	B	C	D
					52)	A	B	C	D	79)	A	B	C	D

80)	A	B	C	D	107)	A	B	C	D	134)	A	B	C	D
81)	A	B	C	D	108)	A	B	C	D	135)	A	B	C	D
82)	A	B	C	D	109)	A	B	C	D	136)	A	B	C	D
83)	A	B	C	D	110)	A	B	C	D	137)	A	B	C	D
84)	A	B	C	D	111)	A	B	C	D	138)	A	B	C	D
85)	A	B	C	D	112)	A	B	C	D	139)	A	B	C	D
86)	A	B	C	D	113)	A	B	C	D	140)	A	B	C	D
87)	A	B	C	D	114)	A	B	C	D	141)	A	B	C	D
88)	A	B	C	D	115)	A	B	C	D	142)	A	B	C	D
89)	A	B	C	D	116)	A	B	C	D	143)	A	B	C	D
90)	A	B	C	D	117)	A	B	C	D	144)	A	B	C	D
91)	A	B	C	D	118)	A	B	C	D	145)	A	B	C	D
92)	A	B	C	D	119)	A	B	C	D	146)	A	B	C	D
93)	A	B	C	D	120)	A	B	C	D	147)	A	B	C	D
94)	A	B	C	D	121)	A	B	C	D	148)	A	B	C	D
95)	A	B	C	D	122)	A	B	C	D	149)	A	B	C	D
96)	A	B	C	D	123)	A	B	C	D	150)	A	B	C	D
97)	A	B	C	D	124)	A	B	C	D					
98)	A	B	C	D	125)	A	B	C	D					
99)	A	B	C	D	126)	A	B	C	D					
100)	A	B	C	D	127)	A	B	C	D					
101)	A	B	C	D	128)	A	B	C	D					
102)	A	B	C	D	129)	A	B	C	D					
103)	A	B	C	D	130)	A	B	C	D					
104)	A	B	C	D	131)	A	B	C	D					
105)	A	B	C	D	132)	A	B	C	D					
106)	A	B	C	D	133)	A	B	C	D					

XXXXXXXXXXXXXXX
XXXXXXXXXXXXXXX
XXXXXXXXXXXXXXX
XXXXXXXXXXXXXXX

Scoring Sheet 12
Tear out for easy use

1)	A	B	C	D	26)	A	B	C	D	53)	A	B	C	D
2)	A	B	C	D	27)	A	B	C	D	54)	A	B	C	D
3)	A	B	C	D	28)	A	B	C	D	55)	A	B	C	D
4)	A	B	C	D	29)	A	B	C	D	56)	A	B	C	D
5)	A	B	C	D	30)	A	B	C	D	57)	A	B	C	D
6)	A	B	C	D	31)	A	B	C	D	58)	A	B	C	D
7)	A	B	C	D	32)	A	B	C	D	59)	A	B	C	D
8)	A	B	C	D	33)	A	B	C	D	60)	A	B	C	D
9)	A	B	C	D	34)	A	B	C	D	61)	A	B	C	D
10)	A	B	C	D	35)	A	B	C	D	62)	A	B	C	D
11)	A	B	C	D	36)	A	B	C	D	63)	A	B	C	D
12)	A	B	C	D	37)	A	B	C	D	64)	A	B	C	D
13)	A	B	C	D	38)	A	B	C	D	65)	A	B	C	D
14)	A	B	C	D	39)	A	B	C	D	66)	A	B	C	D
15)	A	B	C	D	40)	A	B	C	D	67)	A	B	C	D
16)	A	B	C	D	41)	A	B	C	D	68)	A	B	C	D
17)	A	B	C	D	42)	A	B	C	D	69)	A	B	C	D
18)	A	B	C	D	43)	A	B	C	D	70)	A	B	C	D
19)	A	B	C	D	44)	A	B	C	D	71)	A	B	C	D
20)	A	B	C	D	45)	A	B	C	D	72)	A	B	C	D
21)	A	B	C	D	46)	A	B	C	D	73)	A	B	C	D
22)	A	B	C	D	47)	A	B	C	D	74)	A	B	C	D
23)	A	B	C	D	48)	A	B	C	D	75)	A	B	C	D
24)	A	B	C	D	49)	A	B	C	D	76)	A	B	C	D
25)	A	B	C	D	50)	A	B	C	D	77)	A	B	C	D
					51)	A	B	C	D	78)	A	B	C	D
					52)	A	B	C	D	79)	A	B	C	D

80)	A	B	C	D	107)	A	B	C	D	134)	A	B	C	D
81)	A	B	C	D	108)	A	B	C	D	135)	A	B	C	D
82)	A	B	C	D	109)	A	B	C	D	136)	A	B	C	D
83)	A	B	C	D	110)	A	B	C	D	137)	A	B	C	D
84)	A	B	C	D	111)	A	B	C	D	138)	A	B	C	D
85)	A	B	C	D	112)	A	B	C	D	139)	A	B	C	D
86)	A	B	C	D	113)	A	B	C	D	140)	A	B	C	D
87)	A	B	C	D	114)	A	B	C	D	141)	A	B	C	D
88)	A	B	C	D	115)	A	B	C	D	142)	A	B	C	D
89)	A	B	C	D	116)	A	B	C	D	143)	A	B	C	D
90)	A	B	C	D	117)	A	B	C	D	144)	A	B	C	D
91)	A	B	C	D	118)	A	B	C	D	145)	A	B	C	D
92)	A	B	C	D	119)	A	B	C	D	146)	A	B	C	D
93)	A	B	C	D	120)	A	B	C	D	147)	A	B	C	D
94)	A	B	C	D	121)	A	B	C	D	148)	A	B	C	D
95)	A	B	C	D	122)	A	B	C	D	149)	A	B	C	D
96)	A	B	C	D	123)	A	B	C	D	150)	A	B	C	D
97)	A	B	C	D	124)	A	B	C	D					
98)	A	B	C	D	125)	A	B	C	D					
99)	A	B	C	D	126)	A	B	C	D					
100)	A	B	C	D	127)	A	B	C	D					
101)	A	B	C	D	128)	A	B	C	D					
102)	A	B	C	D	129)	A	B	C	D					
103)	A	B	C	D	130)	A	B	C	D					
104)	A	B	C	D	131)	A	B	C	D					
105)	A	B	C	D	132)	A	B	C	D					
106)	A	B	C	D	133)	A	B	C	D					

XXXXXXXXXXXXXX
XXXXXXXXXXXXXX
XXXXXXXXXXXXXX
XXXXXXXXXXXXXX

Secrets To Reducing Exam Stress

What is Stress

Stress is a normal physical response to events that make you feel threatened or upset your balance in some way, such as situations beyond your control.

The body reacts to these situations with physical, mental, and emotional responses that all merge to create what is known as stress.

When you sense danger or events beyond your control the body's defense mechanisms kick into high gear causing a built in chain reaction of events to occur. This is natural for all of us.

Remember the first time someone reprimanded you for something you had done wrong? Not necessarily a parent or relative, but someone in school or at your place of employment where you felt threatened and began feeling stressed and nervous? That was a natural reaction to a set of circumstances that caused you to feel the effects of stress.

This can be a good thing during an emergency or other event but can also be a bad thing when you are trying to concentrate or think clearly for long periods of time, such as during an exam.

What Causes Stress and Anxiety

Stress is caused by fear, plain and simple. The fear of the unknown. The fear of failing. The fear of being unprepared. The fear of loss. The fear of an uncontrollable situation.

Anything beyond our control can cause fear or a sense of danger and this causes the body to release stress hormones, thus increasing your stress and anxiety level.

There are other factors that cause stress too including family, income, job, friends, life situations and others but the main focus of this book is stress directly attributed to exam preparation and taking an exam.

Once you learn how to reduce and manage stress for an exam you can certainly expand its uses to other areas of your life as well. As a matter of fact, I highly recommend that you do. The facts are clear, the less stress you have in your life the longer you will live and the better quality of life you will have.

What Are The Side Effects Of Stress

When stress is not controlled it can cause a significant amount of problems for people taking an exam. You have likely already experienced some of the side effects of stress including:

• Memory Problems

• Lack of Concentration

• Poor Judgement

• Negative Thoughts

• Headaches

• High Blood Pressure

• Upset Stomach

Each of these side effects can affect your exam preparation efforts and performance. As a matter of fact, in some extreme cases it can cause people to "lock up" and have difficulty even taking an exam. These cases are rare but they do exist. If you suffer from this type of reaction you know all too well how difficult it is to perform under these conditions, let alone excel or perform well enough to earn a passing grade.

So how can you control or minimize the effects of stress and even make it work for you?

Learn to Relax

Setting your mind at ease and learning how to relax can reduce stress dramatically. This is much easier said than done, however, there are different techniques to help you relax and each have there own set of benefits.

There are many different ways to relax your mind and body. Some are more difficult than others. Let's begin with an easy way to reduce even the most sever cases of stress.

Slow Breathing

When you begin to feel the effects of stress your breathing accelerates and your heart rate quickens. This is caused by adrenaline being pumped into your system from the body's reaction to a circumstance or situation.

The first thing you have to do is recognize that you are experiencing stress. After you have done that, the easiest and fastest way to reduce your stress level is to slow your breathing.

If you have ever watched a sporting event you have probably seen top athletes using this method to slow their heart rate, reduce adrenaline flow, relax their muscles, and clear their minds.

This helps them think more clearly, react more rapidly, and perform at a higher level. This is exactly what you want to do.

Top athletes do this when adrenaline is not a good thing and can effect performance.

A good example of this is golf. A golfer relies heavily on muscle memory to produce accurate and consistent golf shots. When adrenaline is introduced into their system, say during the final round of a tournament, it can cause a variation in the distance they hit the ball.

This can make them inconsistent at the very time when they need to be the most consistent.

And at the same time... with the stress level now amped up it can cause a player who normally makes sound decisions to now make questionable ones. This is strikingly similar to an exam situation.

Give this method a try. Take a deep breath and exhale slowly. Repeat this several times until your muscles are totally relaxed and your heart rate slows.

Use this method before studying and prior to and during the exam itself! It will help you think more clearly and be able to recall learned information more rapidly. This technique should be the first thing you do when you start to feel anxious or stressed.

"SOMETIMES WHEN PEOPLE ARE UNDER STRESS THEY HATE TO THINK, AND IT'S THE TIME THEY MOST NEED TO THINK."

PRESIDENT BILL CLINTON

Meditation

Please don't be intimidated by the word "meditation". It is not something to fear, rather something to embrace once you know a little more about it.

Meditation can give your mind a chance to take a much needed break, to "shut down", relax and recharge.

The biggest misconception about meditation is that it is something complex. It isn't. It is simply the process of relaxing your mind and body to give it a much needed break. This is exactly what you need to relieve stress.

Time to Meditate

Meditation does not take that long to do and it can be immensely valuable for your mind, body, and spirit. Scheduling a time to meditate is the best way to make sure it happens on a regular basis.

Set aside ten minutes prior to your scheduled study time each day to meditate. This will get you into the routine of doing it. Also schedule ten to twenty minutes prior to taking an exam to meditate when possible. It will help you relax and open your mind for better memory retention during study time and better information recall during exam time.

Meditation Exercises

Follow these simple steps to enjoy a deeper sense of relaxation.

• Sit in a relaxed position.

• Close your eyes.

• Rest your hands, palms up, on your lap.

• Breathe slowly and slightly deeper than normal.

- Concentrate on your breath coming in and going out.

- Quiet your mind. If you are thinking of something try to release the thought and concentrate on breathing again.

- As you become relaxed repeat a calming word or phrase such as "I feel calm" or "I can achieve", or even "I am the best".

- After ten minutes open your eyes slowly.

This should thoroughly relax you and give you positive thoughts and energy. Now your mind is free to accept new information when studying and ready to recall learned information more rapidly and accurately when taking an exam.

Meditation is nothing more than focused relaxation for the mind and body. Look at it this way. You rest your body six to eight hours per night. Sometimes your mind is resting but not always. So your mind doesn't get as much rest as your body does, just as everything else, it needs rest to be able to perform at a high level.

This is good for daily use, but *ultra* effective prior to exam preparation and before an actual exam.

Set Up A Routine

One of the most important actions you can take to reduce stress and anxiety is set up a study routine.

By setting up a regular study routine you remove the stress of trying to find time everyday to study. Schedule the time in advance. Commit to it and stick to it.

You know what time you have to go to work everyday... right? Why not know what time you are going to study everyday? All good habits are scheduled and repeated. Study time should be no different.

Scheduling

The best time to lay out a schedule is about a month to forty five days prior to an exam when possible. All exams are different but mapping out a consistent plan is essential. This is your way to say "this is important to me".

This will give you enough time to review all the material in a timely manner without cramming it all in at the last minute. This alone will reduce your stress level significantly as well as boost your confidence.

How Often Should You Study

A good study routine should consist of regularly scheduled short periods of uninterrupted and focused study time every day. This will give you time to absorb the information when you are alert and can concentrate fully.

Your study time should not consist of hours upon hours of study time in one day and then no study time for several days. This will wear you down and reduce your ability to retain and recall information.

The last minute "all nighter" is the worst thing you can do! This time should only be for a last minute review of the most difficult material.

Plodding through hundreds of pages of information the night before an exam will only deprive you of sleep you desperately need and dilute any information you have already committed to memory.

You might occasionally "luck out" on an exam this way but keep in mind how much better you could have done had you prepared the right way.

How Long Should You Study

The ideal daily study time is an hour to two hours per day maximum! This will ultimately depend on your work, home, family, or school schedule of course but try to arrange something as close to this as possible.

If you schedule four to five hours or more in one day you are most likely defeating the purpose and wasting your time as your retention will start to decrease in hours three and beyond.

This is specially true if you have other commitments that require your time. Scheduling three or more hours of study time per day can actually add MORE stress to your life and reduce your sleeping time.

Either way this is exactly what you want to avoid at all costs! And I do mean ALL COSTS!

Scheduling time each day will keep you mentally fresh and absorbing good information PLUS it will give you the proper time for other commitments too! The outcome... reduce stressed.

Study With A Buddy

Whenever possible try to study with a buddy. Each person brings a different perspective to the learning process. This is a good way to retain new information because you are more focused on the task at hand when you are with someone else.

Plus, when you commit to study with a buddy the chances are you will actually follow through with your scheduled study time. No one likes to break a promise or commitment.

Commitment

Committing to study with a buddy is kind of like working out. It is hard to get motivated and push yourself to workout daily by yourself. That is just a fact. Only the most disciplined people can do this on their own and even some times they find it a challenge.

When you commit to meet a friend to workout it is much easier to keep your routine and commitment. Even though you may not want to workout that day, you recall the commitment you made to your friend and off you go to follow up on your commitment.

That commitment actually carries a lot of psychological weight with it. That is why people follow through with commitments made to others or in public and why it is important for you to commit to study with a buddy.

Plus the company never hurts either. Chances are you will both motivate each other to do more than you would have done alone.

The more you feel that you are not "in this alone" the more relaxed and confident you will be and the more you will get done.

*Note: **IMPORTANT*****Study with a positive minded person. Don't get stuck listening to negative people and their excuses why they can't do this or that. These people are always looking to drag other people "down to their level" and are always reluctant to change to better themselves.*

If you arrange to study with a buddy and the person starts making negative comments... get out now! Don't waist your time trying to bring them up or convert them to your way of thinking.... it won't work! Stay positive and spend your time studying... not counseling. Leave that to the professionals.

Develop Your Concentration

Concentration is described as "intense mental application; complete attention".

It is your minds ability to focus on the task at hand and block out all other influences and distractions. To concentrate on one thing and one thing exclusively... the exam.

Information Retention

Your ability to concentrate is vital to your exam success. The more you concentrate on the subject materials the better you will retain and recall the information when the time comes to perform.

When you concentrate solely on the material it allows you less time to worry about other "stressors" or to give time for negative thoughts to enter in. And negative thoughts will try to work their way in. Self doubt is something that can be destructive so don't give your mind an opportunity to entertain negative thoughts.

For you to perform your best, all attention must be on the study material and the exam. This deep level of concentration will help you maximize your study time. In most cases, the better you can concentrate during your study time the less study time you will actually have to schedule. The saying "quality over quantity" applies to exam preparation too!

I mean... really, who wants to study for 5 hours at one sitting when you can study for 2 hours, with a high level of concentration and focus, and get the same results. No one. **Study Smarter, Not Longer!**

Benefits

Training your mind to concentrate on the task at hand will keep positive thoughts flowing and block out negative thoughts. Think of your mind as a bowl. You can only put so much in a bowl. So the more positive thoughts you put into the bowl the less room there is for negative ones.

Some of the benefits of increasing your level of concentration included:

• Peace of mind

• Self confidence

• Inner strength

• Ability to focus your mind

• Increased memory

• Ability to study and comprehend more quickly

• Less study time

Exercises

Here are some exercises to help you develop your concentration.

1) Select one thought and concentrate on it for ten minutes. This will be difficult at first but the more you do it the easier it will be to block out all other thoughts and concentrate on the one thought you have chosen.

2) Count the words in a paragraph. Count them again to ensure accuracy. Once you have completed this, count several paragraphs and then an entire page.

3) Take an object such as a spoon, fork, or anything out of a drawer. Try to concentrate on the object without mentally describing the object in words. Just focus on the object from all directions.

4) Draw a circle and color it in with any color. Now focus on the object and try not to think of any words, just focus on the object for several minutes.

5) Lie down and relax all your muscles. Once you are completely relaxed concentrated on your heartbeat and imagine your blood flowing throughout your body. After several minutes you should be able to feel the blood moving through your veins.

6) Watch the second hand on a clock. Focus just on the second hand and nothing else. Do this for two to three minutes and fight off the urge to let any other thoughts interfere with your concentration.

7) Close your eyes and visualize the number one. Say the number "one" in your head once you visualize it clearly. Now let it go and focus on the number two and repeat the process up to ten.

8) Take a coin out of your pocket. Relax every muscle in your body and concentrate on the coin and only the coin. View everything about it, its shape, color, material makeup nicks, words. Now close your eyes and visualize the coin in full detail. If you can not visualize the coin in full detail open your eyes and try again.

9) Sit in a chair and relax. Focus on a spot on the wall and release all other thoughts from your mind. Now while looking at the spot on the wall focus on your breathing. Breath in slowly and then exhale slowly. Do this for several minutes.

10) Read an article in the newspaper. Capture the essentials of the article. Now describe the article in as few words as possible to a friend or just aloud to yourself.

Learning to concentrate fully on the task at hand is difficult but the benefits are enormous. It is easy to let your mind wander off and loose your train of thought during an exam.

The better your concentration is during your exam preparation the better your exam scores will be. It is as simple as that.

Concentration is critical, specially towards the end of the exam when it is easy to get distracted and lose focus as you start to get tired.

This is when this training will pay off. You <u>will</u> remain focused and keep your concentration though the entire exam.

Note: IMPORTANT**** *These exercises are not for everyone, however, they are a valuable tool when learning to increase your concentration and mental focus.*

Try to do the exercises every other day. You will notice an increase in your information retention and recall. Plus this will help you study more efficiently and effectively!

Power of Positive Thinking

Positive thinking can reduce stress, improve your overall health, and make you much more interesting and fun to be around.

Although it is unclear exactly why positive thinkers experience health benefits, one of the theories is it helps them deal with stressful situations better. They are thinking of the best outcome, not the worst outcome, and this creates less stress and anxiety. This is better for the mind and the body.

I'll never forget an acquaintance of mine way back in the mid 80's who would shoot down new ideas like clay pigeons. Whenever a new idea would come up he would spend three times the intellectual effort to shoot it down than to consider if it would ever work. In his eyes "it would never work" no matter what it was.

Does that guy sound familiar to you? My guess is he probably does. You might have one or several people like this in your life right now. The best thing you can do is run... run... run.

I have nothing against shooting holes in a new idea to see if it stands the test of scrutiny, but just to dismiss a new idea because it represents change is unhealthy.

Negative people will try with all their might to bring you down. To make you surrender your positive "can do" attitude and keep them company in their pool of negativity. Don't let them!

Glass Half Full or Empty

Are you a "glass half full" or "glass half empty" type of person? Answering this question is a good way to find out if you are an optimist or a pessimist.

If you always see the good side of things (glass half full) then you are an optimist. If not, then you are a pessimist.

Optimists (or positive people) always consider the "what if it could work" side of things. They are happy and easy with a smile. They give as much positive energy as they get from others and are usually interesting and fun to be around.

An optimist is more likely to be successful too. They "will their self to victory". They tell THEMSELVES they can do something and this starts the ball of positivity and success rolling. Just as a snowball rolling down a mountain starts small, once it gains momentum there is little way to stop it.

Self Talk

Why is self talk important? Well, the mind is always thinking and creating "self-talk". Self-talk is the endless stream of thoughts that run through your head.

Self-talk is based on information, reason, logic, and prior experience. Self-talk also comes from misconceptions created because of misinformation or lack of information. This can be negative or positive, depending on your outlook.

For example, if someone asked you to jump over a hurdle and you've never jumped over a hurdle before, your mind would tell you either "you can do this" or "no way you can do this". This is commonly referred to as self-talk.

"PROGRAM THE VOICE INSIDE YOUR HEAD. IT WILL LISTEN, YOU OWN IT."

Programing your self talk will help you control the way you look at things and the attitude you have towards them. Self-talk is enormously powerful and you want to have it on your side.

A good example of the power of self-talk became apparent to me while working out several years ago and its power and control made a lasting impression on me.

In 1998 I started to lap swim at the local YMCA. I started to lap swim for several reasons. First, to lose weight that had accumulated over years of sitting behind a desk and remaining inactive. And second, to relieve some of the stress that comes with an upper level management job that I had been promoted to several years before.

The process of building up to a meaningful workout was slow at first, only a swimming a few laps per session. But over time I had built up to swimming 27 laps (which equalled 3/4 of a mile) per session.

I stayed at that level for many years, mainly because I could get my workout in over an hour long lunch break. But a funny thing happened several years ago when I finally went to work for myself. And it was all brought to light while talking to fellow lap swimmer at the local YMCA.

Through conversation she asked "how far do you swim each day". I said "3/4 of a mile". She asked, "why don't you just swim a mile"? "I don't know" I replied. "I have been doing this for years and never gave it much thought".

The next time in the pool I tried to swim a mile (36 laps) and around lap number twenty my mind began telling me I was tired and it was almost time to quit.

And sure enough, at lap twenty seven I was in no position to go any further. I was done. My mind had convinced my body that 3/4 of a mile was enough for today.

It was hard to believe that my body just started to feel exhausted around the 3/4 mile mark, knowing full well I could swim more laps. So the next day I decided to control my self-talk and tell myself "I am going to swim thirty six laps today" and "I could do anything I put my mind to". I was literally trying to trick myself into thinking I could swim a full mile.

Swimming a full mile was not a problem that day because my mind was reinforcing the belief that I could swim a mile. By controlling my self-talk and keeping the self-talk positive instead of negative I was able to control the outcome and achieve more than what my mind had previously programed me to accept as my unconscious limit.

I have also used this technique to swim two miles in one session and lose over 60 lbs. Controlling your self-talk is powerful, and it works.

Unconscious Limits

Your mind sets unconscious limits for everything that you do based on previous experience and other inputs of information such as things you read or discuss with others. Your mind processes all this information to set predetermined limits for you.

This was exceptionally powerful when world class runners were trying to break the four minute mile mark. It was generally thought that no one could ever run a mile under four minutes.

And for years no one could surpass that mark until May 6th, 1954. Sir Roger Bannister ran a mile in 3:59. Until that day no one had ever recorded running a mile under four minutes.

How strong was that unconscious limit? So strong that it only took ***46 days*** for the record to be broken. The unconscious limit had been stripped away, and in only 46 days another runner achieved what only one man had ever achieved before. The sub four minute mile.

The same applies to your exam preparation. Remove your unconscious limits and give your mind the freedom to perform the way it is capable of. Learning to channel self-talk in a positive direction can help you achieve more than you ever imagined.

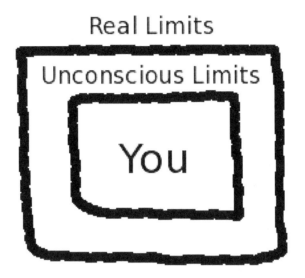

Train Your Mind

In the end, the mind will do what you train it to do. For example, do you ever catch yourself saying subconsciously that you *can't* do something? Of course you have. We all have. That is because we haven't trained our minds to accept the challenge of the task we want to perform.

It is our job to change the way we think. Think positive thoughts. "I CAN do this". "I am the best". "I will pass the exam". Train your mind to think positively and this will reduce your stress level and give you a confident feeling going into the exam.

Do not let others, or your surroundings, dictate your mental state of mind. YOU have the ultimate control and YOU control whether you think positive or negative thoughts.

This takes time and it is something that should be practiced daily. Do not think you can think positive once and everything will occur as you would like it. It just doesn't work that way. Even when you fail, resist the urge to be negative. Everything worthwhile takes some effort. But over time this will work in your favor.

You have to remember you are potentially trying to undo years of "I CAN"T" programming. Years of people telling you "YOU CAN'T" and "NO" and "IT WILL NEVER WORK".

Those are powerful messages built in to your mind. We have all heard them for many years and now is the time to turn it around.

The first "YES I CAN", and "I CAN DO WHATEVER I PUT MY MIND TO" will begin the change. It will start the little snowball rolling down the mountain... and with a little momentum comes massive change!

Self Confidence

Confidence shows in everything you do. From how you look at life to how you treat others. Confident people are people who take action. Confident people are the "doers" in the world. The people who look for ways for things to work rather than look for ways for things to fail.

Confidence is not arrogance. Confidence comes from taking decisive action and not from the outcome of that action. Confident people do not shy away from taking action because they are afraid of a failed outcome. They take action and are undaunted by the prospect of failure.

Arrogance, however, is exactly the opposite. Arrogance does not come from taking action, it comes from the result of the action. Arrogance highlights achievements and hides failures never learning anything from either.

An arrogant person is defined, in their own mind, by both their accomplishments and failures and will shy away from taking action because of the prospect of failure.

Developing Confidence

Confidence is developed through a series of "wins" or "achievements". It is developed through facing your fears and overcoming them. This gives you strength and confidence in your ability to overcome. The more you overcome, the more confident you become.

So how do you build confidence in your ability to pass an exam? Simple.... preparation! Face your fears head on and take action. Prepare every day until you know you are going to pass... there is not doubt!

Review the study material over and over again and build your level of confidence. There is no substitute for hard work and hard work builds confidence.

Have you ever seen a person walk into a room and everyone pays attention? They have a certain confidence about them that radiates form within.

They are not the wealthiest in the room. Nor the most attractive person. But this inner confidence puts them at ease when everyone else may be timid or afraid to step out of their comfort zone.

Confidence and the Exam

Your confidence will have a direct effect on your exam results. If you are confident in your ability to pass the exam it lowers your stress level and opens your mind for clearer thinking. When you project confidence your body reacts differently to circumstances. It gives you the calmness to perform at a high level.

Confidence only comes through preparation. The more you prepare, the more confident you will be in your ability to ace your exam.
This is the type of confidence you must have when you walk into the exam. An undeniable belief that you will pass the exam because of your preparation, determination, and hard work.

Nothing will stand in your way from achieving your goal!

"YOU GAIN STRENGTH, COURAGE AND CONFIDENCE BY EVERY EXPERIENCE IN WHICH YOU STOP TO LOOK FEAR IN THE FACE. YOU ARE ABLE TO SAY TO YOURSELF, 'I HAVE LIVED THROUGH THIS HORROR. I CAN TAKE THE NEXT THING THAT COMES ALONG.' YOU MUST DO THE THING YOU THINK YOU CANNOT DO."

ELEANOR ROOSEVELT

Sleep and Nutrition

The final piece of the puzzle to reducing stress is proper sleep and nutrition. Your body and mind can only function at its highest level if you give it proper rest and proper nutrition (fuel).

Your body and mind needs time to rest and good food to perform. This is easy to overlook and many times it is the first thing you sacrifice when you are preparing for an exam.

You can do everything else right to reduce stress and prepare for an exam but failing to get proper rest and nutrition could cause it all to go to waste.

Once you think about it you can see why these are essential ingredients (no pun intended) to successful exam preparation.

Sleep

Why is sleep so important? Because it is the only time your body has a chance to recharge.

A good sleep regiment should consist of at least six hours of sleep each night so your body and mind are fresh and ready to go the next morning. Anything less an you will not be fully rested and your performance will suffer because of it.

Stress can also impact sleep patterns to a point that is unhealthy. Stress related sleep disorders are fairly common and can have a major impact on your exam performance.

How many times have you tried to solve work or family related problems well into the night. Sometimes it just cannot be avoided but trying to leave work at work and going to bed with a clear mind will leave you refreshed and ready to tackle the problems of the day when the next day arrives.

To get a better nights sleep try these simple tips to reduce stress and rest up.

1) List problems bothering you with possible solutions before bed.

2) Put work into perspective. When work is over, leave it. Turn it off.

3) Designate cell free time. Even if it is only a half hour or during dinner.

4) Never check work email before bed.

5) Try to simplify one thing each day.

6) Grab a nap if you can. Sleep reduces stress hormones.

7) Laugh! Laughter reduces stress and raises <u>anti-stress</u> hormones making it easier to fall asleep.

8) Owning a pets can significantly lower your heart rate and blood pressure letting you rest longer.

9) Hug a family member. Affection reduces stress and makes it easier to sleep.

10) Take a fifteen minute walk. Exercise is the <u>BEST</u> stress reliever and you will be ready to sleep when the time comes!

These tips can make it easier to get a good nights rest and ready to go in the morning.

Nutrition

Proper nutrition to reduce stress you say? Yes, it's true! Proper nutrition plays a key role in our body's performance and ability to rest.

There is plenty of information about the ties between nutrition and sleep. One of my favorite articles is called "Sleep Deeper with Better Nutrition". It covers a mound of information about protein "super foods" and herbs that will help you get a better nights rest naturally.

Some of the "super foods" are items such as green tea, buffalo, walnuts, sardines, artichokes, kiwis, dark chocolate, cherries, and many others. These foods supply the body with super fuel and burn very efficiently so you don't feel full or tired after eating them.

I prefer making adjustments to diet over prescription drugs or other methods because it is natural and enhances the body's ability to rest.

Food or drink that contain sugar or caffeine can give you a temporary boost but the crash won't help you towards the end of the exam when you typically need it the most so try to avoid these.

What If I Fail?

The most successful people fail all the time! It is a result of taking action. There is no shame in failure, only shame in not getting back up, learning from your mistakes, and trying again.

Golf legend Jack Nicklaus used to welcome a bad golf hole or two each round because the sooner he got them out of the way the sooner he could move on and make the round a great one. He embraced temporary failure as part of being successful.

Truthfully, the more you fail the closer you are to succeeding as long as you learn from your mistakes. Few people succeed without failing many times first. It's a learning process and failure is one of the steps. You can say failure is the downpayment on success and it really is. Chances are good you will fail before you succeed but don't let it define you or hold you back. Expect it and learn from it. If you don't fail it shows you haven't taken action and just sat on the sidelines and that is the worst fate of all.

Overcome your fear of failure and success will be yours. Nothing will stand in your way. Preparation is the key. If you have prepared properly you will not fail. But if you should, embrace it, be accountable for it, and start again with more resolve than ever.

The highway is littered with people who have failed. Everyone fails. The people who win get right back on the horse and start riding again.

"I HAVE NOT FAILED. I'VE JUST FOUND 10,000 WAYS THAT WON'T WORK."

THOMAS EDISON

Getting Help

Is there a certain section of material that is just not making sense or sinking in? GET HELP! Don't wait or, worse yet, be too shy to ask for help. Search out help as fast as you can. Now is not the time to be shy or hesitate to ask for assistance.

Many teachers and instructors are more than willing to give you a helping hand. That is their profession and most of them generally love to help people. Take advantage of their help if you need it.

REMEMBER, YOU ARE NOT IN THIS ALONE!

Reaching out for help and getting it will give you a feeling of accomplishment and confidence. That confidence will be your friend and something you want to continually build upon as you ready yourself for your exam.

"ONE IMPORTANT KEY TO SUCCESS IS SELF-CONFIDENCE. AN IMPORTANT KEY TO SELF- CONFIDENCE IS PREPARATION."

ARTHUR ASHE

Common Anatomical Terminology

Anatomy terminology can seem complex and overwhelming when just starting out. Once you familiarize yourself with some of the more common terms it will make your preparation much easier. Just like anything else, it will take practice. Learn and few terms each day and before you know it you will have established a good base to work from.

Take time to familiarize yourself with these terms to make you a better medical coder.

Anatomy Terminology - Number	
Term	**Meaning**
mono-, uni-	one
bi	two
tri	three

Anatomy Terminology - Direction and Position

Term	Meaning
ab-	away from
ad-	toward
ecto-, exo-	outside
endo-	inside
epi-	upon
anterior or ventral	at or near the front surface of the body
posterior or dorsal	at or near the real surface of the body
superior	above
inferior	below
lateral	side
distal	farthest from center
proximal	nearest to center

Anatomy Terminology - Basic Terms

Term	Meaning
abdominal	abdomen
buccal	cheek
cranial	skull
digital	fingers and toes
femoral	thigh
gluteal	buttocks
hallux	great toe
inguinal	groin
lumbar	lowest part of spine
mammary	breast
nasal	nose
occipital	back of head
pectoral	breastbone
thoracic	chest
umbilical	navel
ventral	belly

Anatomy Terminology - Conditions - Prefixes

Term	Meaning
ambi-	both
dys-	bad, painful, difficult
eu-	good, normal
homo-	same
iso-	equal, same
mal-	bad, poor

Anatomy Terminology - Conditions - Suffixes

Term	Meaning
-algia	pain
-emia	blood
-itis	inflammation
-lysis	destruction, breakdown
-oid	like
-opathy	disease of
-pnea	breathing

Anatomy Terminology - Surgical Procedures

Term	Meaning
-centesis	puncture a cavity to remove fluid
-ectomy	surgical removal or excision
-ostomy	a new permanent opening
-otomy	cutting into, incision
-opexy	surgical fixation
-oplasty	surgical repair
-otripsy	crushing or destroying

Medical Terminology Prefix, Root, and Suffixes

Being familiar with Medical Terminology prefixes, roots and suffixes are essential for a medical coder. This illustrates how roots, prefixes, and suffixes are used to denote number or size, direction, color, anatomical locations, as well as other meanings.

Medical Terminology - Prefixes and Roots Denoting Number or Size	
Term	**Meaning**
bi-	two
dipl/o	two, double
hemi-	half
hyper-	over or more than usual
hypo-	under or less than usual
iso-	equal, same
macro-	large
megal/o-	enlargement
micro-	small
mono-	one
multi-	many
nulli-	none
poly-	many
semi-	half, partial
tri-	three
uni-	one

Medical Terminology - Roots Denoting Color

Term	Meaning
chlor/o	green
cyan/o	blue
erythr/o	red
leuk/o	white
melan/o	black
xanth/o	yellow

Medical Terminology - Prefixes and Roots Denoting Relative Direction

Term	Meaning
per-	through
peri-	around
post-	behind, after
poster/o	behind
pre-	before, in front of
pro-	before
retr/o	behind, in back of
sub-	under
super-	beyond
supra-	above
syn-	together
trans-	across
ventr/o	belly

Medical Terminology - Roots Denoting Anatomical Location

Term	Meaning
abdomin/o	abdomen
acr/o	extremity
aden/o	gland
angi/o	vessel
arter/i/o	artery
arthr/o	joint
blast/o	embryo
blephar/o	eyelid
bronch/i/o	bronchus
calcane/o	calaneous
cardi/o	heart
carp/o	carpal, wrist
cephal/o	head
cerebr/o	cerebrum
cheil/o	lip
chol/e	bile, gall
chondr/o	cartilage
cocc/i	coccus
col/o	colon
colp/o	vagina

Medical Terminology - Roots Denoting Anatomical Location

Term	Meaning
condyl/o	condyle
core/o, cor/o	pupil
corne/o	cornea
cost/o	ribs
crani/o	cranium
cycl/o	ciliary body
cyst/o	bladder, sac
cyt/o	cell
dactyl/o	fingers or toes
dent/o	tooth
derm/o	skin
dermat/o	skin
duoden/o	duodenum
enter/o	intestine
esophag/o	esophagus
fibr/o	fiber
gangli/o	ganglion
gastr/o	stomach
gingiv/o	gums
gloss/o	tongue

Medical Terminology - Roots Denoting Anatomical Location

Term	Meaning
gynec/o	women
hem/o, hemat/o	blood
hepat/o	liver
hidr/o	sweat
humer/o	humerus
hydr/o	water
hyster/o	uterus
ile/o	ileum
irid/o, ir/o	iris
ischi/o	ischium
jejun/o	jejunum
kerat/o	cornea
lacrim/o	tear
laryng/o	larynx
lip/o	fat
lith/o	stone, calculus
lumb/o	loin, lumbar area
ment/o	chin
my/o	muscle
myel/o	spinal cord, bone marrow

Medical Terminology - Roots Denoting Anatomical Location

Term	Meaning
nas/o	nose
nephr/o	kidney
neur/o	nerve
omphal/o	umbilicus, navel
onych/o	nail
oophor/o	ovary
opthalm/o	eye
orchid/o	testicles
oste/o	bone
ot/o	ear
pancreat/o	pancreas
pely/i	pelvis
peps/o/ia	digestion
phalang/o	phalange
pharyng/o	pharynx
phas/o	speech
phleb/o	veins
pleur/o	pleura
pne/o	air, breathing
pneum/o, pneumono	lung

Medical Terminology - Roots Denoting Anatomical Location

Term	Meaning
pod/o	foot
proct/o	rectum, anus
psych/o	mind
pub/o	pubis
py/o	pus
pyel/o	kidney
rect/o	rectum
ren/o	kidney
retin/o	retina
rhin/o	nose
salping/o	fallopian tube
scler/o	sclera
spermat/o	sperm
splen/o	spleen
stern/o	sternum, breastbone
stomat/o	mouth
thorac/o	thorax, chest
trache/o	trachea
traumat/o	tramua
tympan/o	eardrum

Medical Terminology - Roots Denoting Anatomical Location

Term	Meaning
ur/o	urine
ureter/o	ureter
urethr/o	urethra
vas/o	vessel
viscer/o	gut, contents of the abdomen

Medical Terminology - Other Prefixes

Term	Meaning
a-, an-	without
anti-	against
auto-	self
brady-	slow
con-	with
contra-	against
dis-	free of
dys-	difficult or without pain
mal-	bad, poor
neo-	new
syn-	together
tachy-	fast

Medical Terminology - Other Roots

Term	Meaning
necr/o	dead
noct/i	night
par/o	bear
phag/o	eat
phil/o	attraction
plast/o	repair, formation
pyr/o	fire, fever
scler/o	tough, hard
sinistr/o	left
syphil/o	syphilis
therap/o	treatment
therm/o	heat
thromb/o	thrombosis
troph/o	development

Medical Terminology - Other Suffixes

Term	Meaning
algia	pain
ar	pertaining to
centesis	puncture
clysis	irrigation
ectasia	dilatation, dilation
ectomy	excision
emes/is	vomiting
emia	blood
esthesia	feelings
genesis, gen/o	development, formation, beginning
gnosis	know
ia	noun ending
ia, ic	pertaining to
it is	inflammation
manual	hand
meter	measuring instrument
oid	resembling
ologist	one who studies
ology	study of
oma	tumor

Medical Terminology - Other Suffixes

Term	Meaning
opia	vision
orrhagia	hemorrhage
orrhaphy	suture
orrhea	flow
orrhexis	rupture
osis	condition of
ostomy	new opening
otomy	incision
pedal	foot
pexy	fixing, fixation
phob/ia	fear
plasm	growth
plegia, plegic	paralysis
ptosis	drooping
scope, scopy	examining, looking at
spasm	twitching
sperm	sperm
stasis	slow, stop
tome	instrument
tripsy	crushing

Notes

Notes

Notes

Notes

Resources

Exam Preparation Products We Recommend

Medical Coding Exam Prep Course
http://medicalcodingpro.com/medical-coding-certification-prep-course

Medical Coding Exam System
http://medicalcodingexamsystem.com

Faster Coder - Code Faster - Code Better
http://fastercoder.com

Other Resources

Elite Members Area – 7 day FREE trial!
http://medicalcodingpromembers.com

Medical Coding Pro – main website
http://medicalcodingpro.com

Code Lookup Program - http://www.findacode.com/?pc=MEDCOPRO

MEDICAL CODING PRO

Medical Coding Pro provides information about medical coding. We also help people in the medical coding community prepare for the medical coding certification exam.

Our mission is to help everyone we can pass the exam and gain their certification as quickly as possible.To do this we offer quality exam preparation tools such as Medical Coding Practice Exams, the Medical Coding Exam System, the Medical Coding Exam Strategy and the Medical Coding Pro Elite Members Area.

Visit us on the web at:

www.MedicalCodingPro.com

www.MedicalCodingProMembers.com

www.MedicalCodingExamSystem.com

www.MedicalCodingNews.org

CPSIA information can be obtained
at www.ICGtesting.com
Printed in the USA
BVHW01s0939171018
530410BV00028B/208/P

9 781987 759693